Weight Watchers Instant Pot Freestyle Cookbook 2021

350-Days Easy & New WW Freestyle Recipes to Heal Your Body and Lose Weight Quickly

Evelyn Bittner

Table of Contents

INTRODUCTION

"If you're looking for more information on the Weight Watchers Program then, grab a chair & buckle down, because this is the ebook that you've been looking for."

In the current situation with obesity & the amount of overweight people in the UK & USA, there couldn't be a more important time than now to focus on health issues.

There is a modern stereotype of someone sitting on the couch at home watching the television, with a remote in one hand & a large bag of crisps in the other & a few bowls of snacks on the coffee table beside you.

It seems to be a distant memory of people of all ages out walking or running & children playing sport at their local playing park or sports centre.

So what has changed in recent years?

I think the general perception of keeping fit & healthy has changed & that there isn't enough emphasis put on the subject. The more gadgets that becomes available to people, the more chances of you becoming a couch potato. You just have to look at the types of things that would prevent you from doing exercise - Games Consoles, Satellite TV, Mobile Phones, MP3 & 4 Players... These are the type of things that are causing people, especially the younger generation to stay indoors more often.

Joining a club like Weight Watchers is a huge step in the right direction, as not only will you get involved with a program with a sensible action plan, but you will be getting out of the house & meeting new people with a similar goal to yourself - losing weight & getting fitter.

The new Weight Watchers Freestyle plan, which was launched in the U.S. on 12/3/17, now includes a much wider range of over 200 zero SmartPoints foods from which to base your meals and snacks including eggs, skinless chicken breast, skinless turkey breast, fish and seafood, corn, beans, peas, lentils, tofu, nonfat plain yogurt and so much more.

Previously, only fruits and vegetables had been considered zero points.

While you are always free to eat whatever you want on Weight Watchers, the Freestyle plan nudges you toward choosing nutritious foods by assigning them lower or even zero SmartPoints.

★★ WW INSTANT POT EGGS

Instant Pot Hard Boiled Eggs

Prep Time: 15mins, Cooking Time: 20mins, Serving: 4, Point value: 3

Ingredients

- 16 - large eggs, 1 - cup water

Instructions

1. Spot the wire rack in the base of the Instant Pot. Pour in some water.
2. Spot the crude eggs on the rack and fit them in firmly. I can typically fit 16, yet that will rely upon the extent of your eggs.
3. Close the Instant Pot, ensure the valve is shut and hit the manual catch. Lessen the opportunity to 4 minutes and let them cook.
4. When the clock goes off, hit drop and discharge the weight. Abandoning them in there will result in them overcooking.
5. Exchange them to a huge bowl and spread with virus water. Let cool for 5 minutes.
6. Strip while still warm and flush any shell pieces off.
7. Use promptly or store in the ice chest.

Nutrition Information: Calories 62g, Fat 4g, Carbs g, Sugars 0g, Protein 5g

Instant Pot Hard Boiled Eggs

Prep Time: 10mins, Cook Time: 5mins, Serving: 12, Point value: 2

Ingredients

- 12 - large eggs, 1 - cup water, Ice

Instructions

1. Spot trivet at the base of the internal Instant Pot dish.
2. Spot eggs over trivet, stacking equally if essential.
3. Add some water to the container. Close the cover and set Instant Pot for 5 minutes on Manual at HIGH weight.
4. Enable pot to discharge the weight normally for 5 minutes, at that point in all respects cautiously fast discharge any outstanding steam.
5. Scoop eggs out of pot and spot in an ice shower for 5 minutes.
6. Expel from the ice shower and strip or store in the cooler until prepared to utilize.

Nutrition Information: Calories 71g, Fat 1g, Carbs 3g, Sugar 0.4g, Protein 6g

Instant Pot Egg Bites with Spinach & Prosciutto

Prep Time: 15mins, Cook Time: 10mins, Serving: 2, Point value: 18

Ingredients

- 4 - large eggs
- 3 - ounces finely grated parmesan cheese
- 2 - ounces heavy whipping cream
- ½ - ounce fresh spinach
- ½ - ounce prosciutto
- ½ - teaspoon black pepper
- 1/8 - teaspoon salt

Instructions

1. Utilizing a silicone egg chomps form, uniformly partition the spinach and prosciutto among the 7 shape compartments.
2. In a blending bowl, consolidate eggs, parmesan cheddar, substantial cream, salt, and pepper. Race until well-beaten and smooth.
3. Empty the blend into the form, around 3-4 tablespoons for every compartment, topping off about 80% to the top. Spread firmly with foil.
4. Include 1/2 containers water to the weight cooker pot. Spot the trivet inside. Cautiously lower the shape onto the trivet.
5. Secure and seal the top. Steam for 10 minutes at high weight, trailed by 10 minutes of regular discharge. Physically discharge any residual weight.
6. Reveal and expel the egg nibbles shape from the weight cooker. Dispose of the foil. Alter onto a plate to discharge the egg nibbles.

Nutrition Information: Calories 400g, Fat 29g, Carb 2.5g, Sugars 2g, Protein 27g

Instant Pot Egg Roll Bowls

Prep Time: 5mins, Cook Time: 1min, Servings: 4, Point value: 10

Ingredients

- 1 - lb ground pork
- 1 - bag pre- cole slaw
- ½ - cup bone broth
- 1 - tbsp soy sauce or to taste
- 1 - tbsp garlic powder
- 1 - tbsp ground ginger
- ½ - tsp pepper or to taste
- ½ - tsp salt or to taste
- Wonton Chips
- 1 – pkg. egg roll wrappers
- vegetable or olive oil

Instructions

1. Spot Instant Pot on saute. Hold up until it's warm and after that include pork. Include seasonings and soy sauce and darkish coloured meat. On the off hazard that you are using a lump of lean meat, you may not need to delete it while it is achieved.
2. At the factor when meat is caramelized, turn Instant Pot off and encompass the 1/2 glass bone inventory. Include a % of coleslaw mixture on pinnacle and DO NOT blend. Spot top on and swing cope with to fixing role.
3. Set Instant Pot on manual high weight for 0 mins. On the off chance that you have a extra up to date model Instant Pot, you choose the weight prepare dinner seize rather for zero minutes. What's greater, sure zero minutes is in reality a component.
4. At the point whilst the clock is up, carry out a snappy discharge. At the factor while weight is discharged, open cautiously and give everything a brisk blend.
5. Spoon into dishes and appreciate
6. Preheat broiler to four hundred degrees even as Instant Pot is preheating on saute.
7. Cut egg fold wrappers into strips and shrubbery with olive or veggie oil.
8. Heat in preheated broiler for four-5 mins till bubbly and dark coloured. WATCH those carefully in mild of the reality that they move from darker to fed on brief
9. Give chips a threat to chill and recognize together with your egg flow bowls

Nutrition Information: Calories 230g, Fat 16g, Carbs 6g, Sugars 2g, Protein 15g

Instant Pot Keto Egg Cups on the Run

Prep Time: 5mins, Cook Time: 10mins, Serving: 6, Point value: 5

Ingredients

- 4 - eggs
- 1 - cup diced vegetables such as onions, bell peppers, mushrooms, tomatoes
- ½ - cup shredded sharp cheddar cheese
- ¼ - cup half and half
- Salt and Pepper to taste
- 2 - tablespoons chopped cilantro

For Finishing: ½ - cup shredded cheese of choice

Instructions

1. Spot some water in your Instant Pot, and spot a trivet in the pot.
2. Spot the egg bumps on the trivet.
3. Cook for 5 minutes at a high weight, and rapidly discharge remaining weight.
4. Top with residual 1/2 measure of cheddar, and either cook or spot noticeable all-around fryer for 2-3 minutes, until the cheddar on top is dissolved and daintily seared.

Nutrition Information: Calories 115g, Fat 9g, Carbs 2g, Sugar 1.3g, Protein 9g

Perfect Instant Pot Soft-Boiled Eggs

Prep Time: 2mins, Cook Time: 3mins, Serving: 4, Point value: 4

Ingredients:

- 2 - cups water, 4 - eggs

Instructions

1. Pour some water into the addition of the Instant Pot. Lay the steamer embeds inside. Spot 4 eggs on top.
2. Spread the pot. Utilizing the manual catch, set the pot to 3 minutes and low weight. Ensure the valve on top is set to fixing. Fill a bowl with ice water or cold faucet water.
3. At the point when the 3 minutes are up, which will take increasingly like 9 minutes, change the valve to venting, let the steam escape for close to 1 minute, cautiously evacuate the top to abstain from steaming your face, exchange eggs to water shower, let cool for 30 seconds or thereabouts, at that point strip, season and eat.

Nutrition Information: Calories 106.6g, Fat 1.3g, Carbs 20.8g, Sugars 8.2g, Protein 2.3g

Instant Pot Hard Boiled Eggs

Prep Time: 10mins, Cook Time: 5mins, Serving: 4, Point value: 12

Ingredients

- 4 – Eggs, 1 - cup water, Instant Pot electric pressure cooker

Instructions

1. Pour the water into the pot, and place the eggs in a steamer basket if you have one. If you don't, just use the rack that came with your pot.
2. Close the lid, set for 5 minutes at high pressure.
3. It will take the cooker approximately 5 minutes to build to pressure and then 5 minutes to cook. I let the pressure naturally reduce for an additional 5 minutes after the cooking cycle completed, and then did a quick pressure release. That's around 15 minutes, total.
4. Place the hot eggs into cool water to halt the cooking process. You can peel immediately, or wait– it's up to you.

Nutrition Information: Calories 343g, Fat 8g, Carbs 14g, Sugars 0.4g, Protein 15g

Keto Chicken Enchilada Bowl

Prep Time: 20mins, Cook Time: 30mins, Serving: 4, Point value: 25

Ingredients

- 2 - tablespoons coconut oil
- 1 - pound of boneless, skinless chicken thighs
- ¾ - cup red enchilada sauce
- ¼ - cup water
- ¼ - cup chopped onion
- 1– 4 oz can diced green chilies

Toppings:
- 1 - Whole avocado, diced
- 1 - cup shredded cheese
- ¼ - cup chopped pickled jalapenos
- ½ - cup sour cream
- 1 - Roma tomato

Instructions

1. In a pot or Dutch broiler over medium warmth dissolve the coconut oil. When hot, singe fowl thighs till softly darkish colored.
2. Pour in enchilada sauce and water at that factor includes onion and green chilies. Diminish warmth to a stew and unfold.
3. Cook fowl for 17-25mins or till bird is sensitive and completely cooked thru to in any event one hundred sixty-five levels internal temperature.
4. Carefully evacuates the fowl and notice onto a work floor. Hack or shred chicken at that point encompass it once again into the pot.
5. Let the chicken stew revealed for an extra 10mins to ingest season and permit the sauce to diminish a bit.
6. To serve, pinnacle with avocado, cheddar, jalapeno, acrid cream, tomato, and some others desired garnishes. Don't hesitate to regulate these on your inclination.
7. Serve by myself or over cauliflower rice whenever wanted certainly ensure to refresh your very own nourishment data as required.

Nutrition Information: Calories: 568g, Fat 40.2g, Carbs 10.41g, Sugar 4.2g, Protein 38.38g

No Noodle Instant Pot Lasagna

Prep Time: 10mins, Cook Time: 25mins, Servings: 8, Point value: 16

Ingredients

- 1 - pound ground beef
- 2 - cloves garlic minced
- 1 - small onion
- 1 ½ - cups ricotta cheese
- ½ - cup Parmesan cheese
- 1 - large egg
- 1 - jar marinara sauce 25 ounces
- 8 - ounces mozzarella sliced

Instructions

1. On sauté setting, dark colored the ground hamburger with the garlic and onion.
2. While the meat is sautéing, join the ricotta cheddar with the Parmesan and egg in a little blending bowl.
3. Channel oil and expel meat blend from Instant Pot.
4. In a medium size bowl blend meat blend with 25 ounces container of marinara
5. Next, utilizing a round dish that fits inside your Instant Pot layer half of your lasagna meat, mozzarella and ricotta cheddar blend rehashing for a second time until no fixings remain. Top with ½ c of saved marinara sauce.
6. Spot sling in Instant Pot over the rack and pour in some water.
7. Set dish in moment pot. Spread freely with aluminum foil whenever wanted to shield buildup from trickling on the lasagna.
8. Join cover, close valve, and cook on high weight for 9 minutes.
9. Vent steam, evacuate the cover and serve.

Nutrition Information: Calories 365g, Fat 25g, Carbs 7g, Sugars 4g, Protein 25g

Instant Pot Copy Cat Chipotle Barbacoa

Prep Time: 10mins, Cook Time: 120min, Serving: 4, Point value: 8

Ingredients

- 3 - pounds chuck roast beef
- ½ - cup broth beef, chicken
- 2-4 - chipotle chiles in adobo
- 2 - tablespoon raw apple cider vinegar
- 2 - tablespoon Lemon Juice
- 2 - tablespoon lime juice
- 1 - tablespoon dried or fresh oregano
- 1 - tablespoon cumin
- 3 - garlic cloves

- 2 - Whole bay leaves
- salt and pepper to taste

Instructions

1. Defrost the cooler dinner in your Instant Pot treated steel holder. I like to give mine a chance to be semi-solidified so I don't need to stress over including fluid yet you can likewise defrost totally to abbreviate the cooking time.
2. Next, dump every one of the substances in the spotless holder, Place the moment pot top on the base, close, and afterward ensure the weight valve is fixed. At that point set the Instant Pot to the manual capacity for 120 min.
3. Finally, when all the meat is finished cooking and squeezing gradually open the cover and spread separated the meat with a fork. Take out whatever herb stems are left and now you're prepared to appreciate this delicious formula

Nutrition Information: Calories 242g, Fat 12g, Carbs 9g, Sugars 3g, Protein 31g

Instant Pot Keto Steak Bites

Prep Time: 5mins, Cook Time: 9mins , Serving: 4, Point value: 14

Ingredients

- 2 - lbs stew meat
- 4 - tsp steak seasoning
- ¼ - tsp salt
- 2 - tsp avocado oil
- 2 - tbsp ghee
- 1 - tbsp dried onion flakes
- 1 - clove garlic
- 4 - ounces mushrooms
- ½ - cup bone broth

Instructions

1. Turn on Instant Pot to 'Saute' mode.
2. When warmed, include oil and hamburger stew meat, garlic, and mushrooms and cook a couple of minutes, until seared. Mix as often as possible so the garlic doesn't consume.
3. Include every single residual fixing. Mix to blend well.
4. Close cover and seal valve. Set high weight and cook 9 minutes. Speedy discharge weight

Nutrition Information: Calories 430g, Fat 21.6g, Carbs 4.9g, Sugars 2.3g, Protein 51.5g

Instant Pot Chili Lime Steak Bowl

Prep Time: 8mins, Cook Time: 10mins, Serving: 4, Point value: 13

Ingredients

- 1.2-2 - pounds of fajita steak strips
- 1 - tablespoon of water
- 1 - teaspoon minced garlic
- 1 - tablespoon of EVOO
- 2 - teaspoons of lime juice
- ½ - teaspoon chili powder
- ½ - teaspoon sea salt
- ½ - teaspoon cracked pepper
- 1 - teaspoon of Cholula
- 2-3 Avocado diced

Instructions

1. Turn your IP on sauté and include olive oil.
2. When hot, include garlic and cook until a brilliant shading.
3. At that point include every single outstanding fixing, and blend well with wooden spoon.
4. Spot top on, and put on Manual High Pressure for 10 minutes. Complete a QPR.
5. When weight is discharged, evacuated cover.
6. Turn skillet back onto sauté mode, and work the meat to split it up into little pieces.
7. Keep on sauté mode until fluid has been decreased significantly.
8. Permit to cool and serve in a bowl, and afterward encompass it with your diced avocado. Yum

Nutrition Information: Calories 365g, Fat 17g, Carbs 7g, Sugars 4.6g, Protein 36g

Creamy Salsa Chicken Recipe

Prep Time: 10mins, Cook Time: 20mins, Servings: 6, Point value: 9

Ingredients

- 2.5 - 3 pounds chicken breasts
- ½ - cup chicken broth
- 4 - oz cream cheese
- ½ - cup cottage cheese
- 1 - cup salsa
- 1-2 - tsp taco or fajita seasoning

Instructions

1. Put the bird bosoms and fowl soup in the Instant Pot. Cook at the rooster putting with the vent fixed for 10mins.
2. Watch that the hen is in any occasion one hundred sixty ranges with a meat thermometer.

3. Expel the chicken to a considerable bowl.
4. Spare half of degree of the cooking fluid and dispose of the rest. Include the held cooking fluid and distinct fixings to the Instant Pot.
5. Turn at the Sauté setting. Rush till the cream cheddar and curds have liquefied.
6. Swing to Keep Warm. Shred the hen. Add lower back to the sauce in the Instant Pot.
7. Present with discretionary fixings.

Nutrition Information: Calories 310g, Fat 12g, Carbs 4g, Sugars 2g, Protein 43g

Instant Pot Creamy Garlic Tuscan Chicken Thighs

Prep Time: 5mins, Cook Time: 30mins, Servings: 4, Point value: 9

Ingredients

- 4 - chicken thighs fat
- 4 - oz cream cheese
- 2 ½ - cups fresh spinach
- ¼ - cup sundried tomatoes
- 1 - tbsp Bouillon Chicken
- ¼ - cup parmesan cheese
- 3 - garlic cloves
- 1 - tsp olive oil
- 1 - cup sodium chicken broth
- 1 - cup milk
- 2 - tbsp whipping cream
- 2 - tsp Italian Seasoning
- 1 - tsp cornstarch
- 1 - tsp water
- salt and pepper to taste
- parsley optional for garnish

Instructions

1. Flush the chicken and pat dry. Empty the olive oil into the Instant Pot.
2. Season the fowl with 1 tsp of the Italian Seasoning, salt, and pepper.
3. Spot the Instant Pot on the Sauté capability. Darker the 2 sides of the fowl for 2-3mins
4. Include the bird soup, milk, better than Bouillon and staying Italian Seasoning to the pot.
5. Close the Instant Pot and Seal. Cook on Manual/High-Pressure cooking for 14mins.
6. At the factor when the pot indicates it has completed, snappy discharge the steam.
7. Open the pot and evacuate the chicken.
8. Include the sundried tomatoes, cream cheddar, whipping cream, parmesan Reggiano, garlic, and spinach to the pot.
9. Cook for three-four minutes until the cheddar has liquefied and the spinach has withered.
10. Join the cornstarch and water in a touch bowl. Blend. Add it to the pot.

14

11. This will thicken up the cream sauce.
12. Either adds the hen returned to the pot with the cream sauce or spots the fowl in a serving dish and showers the sauce during.

Nutrition Information: Calories: 226g, Fat 14g, Carbs 6g, Sugar 3.2g, Protein 17g

Instant Pot Chili Verde

Prep Time: 15mins, Cook Time: 25mins, Servings: 4, Point value: 10

Ingredients

- 2 - pounds boneless skinless chicken thighs
- 12 - ounces tomatillos husked and quartered
- 8 - ounces poblano peppers stemmed
- 4 - ounces jalapeño peppers stemmed
- 4 - ounces onions
- ¼ - cup water
- 5 - cloves garlic
- 2 teaspoons ground cumin
- 1 ½ - teaspoons salt

For finishing:
- ¼ - ounce chopped cilantro leaves
- 1 - tablespoon fresh lime juice

Instructions

1. Include tomatillos, poblanos, jalapeños, onions, and water to the weight cooker. Appropriate garlic, cumin, and salt on top. Ultimately, include chicken thighs. Secure and seal the cover. Cook at a high weight for 15 minutes, trailed by a manual weight discharge. Reveal and exchange just the chicken to a cutting board. Cut into nibble estimated pieces. Put aside.
2. Add cilantro and lime juice to the weight cooker. Utilize a submersion blender or ledge blender to puree the blend.
3. Select the saute mode on the weight cooker for medium warmth. Return the chicken to the blend. Bubble for around 10 minutes to thicken the sauce, mixing sporadically. Serve and enhancement with extra cilantro.

Nutrition Information: Calories 310g, Fat 15g, Carb 10g, Sugars 4.5g, Protein 37g

Easy Low Carb Chicken Soup

Prep Time: 20mins, Cooking Time: 15mins, Serving: 2, Point value: 5

Ingredients

- 10 - cups bone broth or chicken stock
- ½ - tsp garlic powder
- ½ - tsp dried oregano
- 1 - cup thinly sliced celery
- 1 ½ - cups diced butternut squash
- 2 - cups jicama
- 4 - cups cooked chicken
- ¼ - cup chopped fresh parsley
- 1 - Tbsp apple cider vinegar
- sea salt and pepper

Instructions

1. Join the juices, garlic powder, dried oregano, celery, butternut squash, and jicama in a substantial pot.
2. Heat to the point of boiling, at that point lower warmth and stew for 30 minutes, or until veggies are fork delicate.
3. Include the chicken and cook for an additional 5 minutes, or until warmed through
4. Expel from the warmth and include the parsley and apple juice vinegar.
5. Season with ocean salt and pepper to taste before serving.

Nutrition Information: Calories: 190g, Fat 5g, Carbs 5g, Sugar 2.1g, Protein 26g

Low Carb Chicken Taco Soup

Prep Time: 8mins, Cook Time: 30mins, Serving: 4, Point value: 16

Ingredients

- 1 - pound chicken breasts
- ½ - cup diced onion
- 4 - cloves garlic, minced
- 1 - tablespoon chipotles in adobo sauce
- 1 - tablespoon cumin
- ½ - teaspoon chili powder
- ½ - teaspoon paprika
- ½ - teaspoon salt
- 2 - tablespoons lemon juice
- 1 - tablespoon lime juice

- 2 - cups chicken broth
- 8 - ounces cream cheese
- ½ - cup chopped cilantro

Instructions

1. Include the chicken, onion, garlic, chipotles, cumin, stew powder, paprika, salt, lemon juice, lime juice, and chicken juices to an Instant Pot.
2. Spread, swing vents to fixing and cook on high weight for 18 minutes.
3. Enable strain to discharge normally, around 10 minutes, before evacuating the cover.
4. Expel chicken from pot and shred with two forks.
5. Turn the Instant Pot to sauté and include the cream cheddar. Whisk always until the cream cheddar is completely softened and joined.
6. Turn Instant Pot off and return chicken to the pot. Include the cilantro and blend well to join.
7. Serve right away

Nutrition Information: Calories: 424g, Fat 25g, Carbs 7g, Sugar 4g, Protein 41g

---

Instant pot Low Carb Buffalo Chicken Soup

Prep Time: 10mins, Cook Time: 20mins, Serving: 1, Point value: 3

Ingredients

- 1 - tbsp Olive oil
- ½ - large Onion
- ½ - cup Celery
- 4 - cloves Garlic
- 1 - lb Shredded chicken
- 4 - cup Chicken bone broth
- 3 - tbsp Buffalo sauce
- 6 - oz Cream cheese
- ½ - cup Half & half

Instructions

1. Press the Saute to catch on the Instant Pot. Include the oil, slashed onion, and celery. Cook for around 5-10 minutes, mixing every so often until onions are translucent and begin to dark colored.
2. Include garlic. Saute for about a moment, until fragrant. Press the Off catch.
3. Include the destroyed chicken, soup, and bison sauce.
4. Spread and seal the Instant Pot. Press the Soup catch and change time to 5 minutes. In the wake of cooking is finished, given weight a chance to discharge normally for 5 minutes, at that point change to fast discharge and open the top.
5. Scoop about a measure of fluid from the edge of the Instant Pot and fill a blender. Include the cubed cream cheddar. Puree until smooth. (On the off chance that it's difficult to mix, you can include somewhat more fluid.)

6. Empty the blend over into the Instant Pot. Include the half and half or overwhelming cream. Blend until smooth.

Nutrition Information: Calories 270g, Fat 16g, Carbs 4g, Sugar 1g, Protein 27g

Loaded Keto Cauliflower Bowl

Prep Time: 20mins, Cooking Time: 15mins, Serving: 4, Point value: 16

Ingredients

- 2 - cups fresh cauliflower
- 3 - tablespoons butter
- ¼ - cup diced onion
- ¼ - cup pickled jalapeno slices
- 2 - cups cooked brisket
- 2 - ounces cream cheese, softened
- 1 - cup shredded sharp cheddar
- ¼ - cup heavy cream
- ¼ - cup cooked crumbled bacon
- 2 - tablespoons sliced green onions

Instructions

1. Slash cauliflower into nibble measure pieces. Steam or cook by means of most loved technique until fork delicate and set side.
2. Set warmth to medium and include margarine, onion, and jalapeno cuts to skillet. Sauté until onions translucent and fragrant.
3. Lessen heat somewhat and include cooked brisket [or decision of extra meat/chicken] and cream cheese. If blend starts to stick or cook too rapidly, diminish heat a bit. Keep cooking until cream cheddar is warmed through and effectively blended.
4. Mood killer heat. Include sharp cheddar, overwhelming cream, and cauliflower. Mix blend rapidly until all cheeses are dissolved and completely joined.
5. Sprinkle with disintegrated bacon, green onions. Serve warm.

Nutrition Information: Calories 329g, Fat 27g, Carbs 5g, Sugar 1.4g, Protein 18g

Low Carb Keto Zuppa Toscana Soup Recipe

Prep Time: 10mins, Cook Time: 30mins, Serving: 1, Point value: 17

Ingredients

- 1 - lb mild Italian sausage
- 1 - bag whole radishes 16 ounces
- 1 - medium onion diced
- 2 - teaspoons minced garlic
- 32 - ounces chicken or vegetable broth
- ⅓ - cup heavy whipping cream

- 2 to 3 - cups kale leaves

Instructions

1. Begin by cutting the radishes into little lumps as found in the photographs. I utilized a sustenance processor. The littler the radishes the faster it cooks.
2. Slice the onion.
3. On medium warmth, dark-colored your wiener in a similar pot you intend to use for the soup.
4. After the hotdog is totally dark colored include the juices, onions, and radishes.
5. Presently include the garlic.
6. Give this cook over medium warmth until the radishes a chance to have completely cooked and are pleasant and delicate.
7. Ultimately, include the overwhelming whipping cream and the kale leaves. Make certain to tear the kale leaves into chomp measure pieces.
8. Cook for a couple of minutes more until the kale leaves are delicate.
9. Serve warm and appreciate!

Nutrition Information: Calories 363.6g, Fat 27.3g, Carbs 12.3g, Sugars 5g, Protein 17.8g

Instant Pot Chicken Zoodle Soup

Prep Time: 10mins, Cook Time: 20mins, Servings: 6, Point value: 5

Ingredients

- 1 - tsp Olive Oil
- 1 - small red onion
- 3 - carrots
- 3 - celery ribs
- 1 - banana pepper
- 1 - jalapeno pepper
- 2 - garlic cloves
- salt and fresh ground pepper
- 1 - bay leaf
- 1 - pound chicken breasts
- 6 - cups \fat free chicken broth
- 2 - tsp apple cider vinegar
- 4 - small zucchini spiralized

Instructions

1. Pour 1 tablespoon of the olive oil within the pot of your weight cooker and heat it over medium-excessive warmth.
2. Include onions, carrots, celery, peppers, and garlic; season with salt and pepper and saute for four to 5 minutes.
3. Include cove leaf and layer the chicken bosoms over the veggies.
4. Blend in chook soup and apple juice vinegar. Spread weight cooker with the top.

5. Begin cooking over again excessive warm temperature till you obtain weight 6mins.
6. Decrease warm temperature and cook dinner at a regular weight for 9mins.
7. Discharge the burden; when venting is completed, expel the duvet and take out the hen; change bird to a slicing board and shred it.
8. Include bird once more into the pot and mix in spiralized zucchini.
9. Cook over medium-excessive warmth for around four minutes, or till noodles are cooked to an excellent floor. Spoon soup into dishes.
10. Shower with STAR Olive Oil with Fresh Rosemary and serve.

Nutrition Information: Calories 164g, Fat 5g, Carbs 10g, Sugars 6g, Protein 19g

Instant Pot Keto Bacon Cheeseburger Soup

Prep Time: 15mins, Cook Time: 15mins, Servings: 6, Point value: 29

Ingredients

- 6 - oz bacon chopped
- 1 ½ - pounds hamburger
- 1 - large onion diced
- 2 - large carrots diced
- 2 - stalks celery diced
- 4 - cups cauliflower chopped
- 4 - cups beef or chicken broth
- 4 - ounces cream cheese
- 1 - cup shredded sharp cheddar cheese or more to taste
- Sea salt will depend on the broth you use, start with a 1/2 teaspoon

Instructions

1. Utilizing the saute element on your Instant Pot, dark-colored your bacon, evacuate
2. Proceed with the ground meat. Darker the meat until cooked through, expel.
3. Include every one of your vegetables, and saute a couple of minutes to diminish (include some coconut oil on the off chance that you utilized a slice of lean meat and there is no fat left in the pot)
4. Pour in the stock.
5. Lock on the cover set manual for 7 minutes.
6. Fast discharge.
7. Presently, utilizing a submersion blender, directly in the pot, puree the vegetables.
8. Mix in the cheeses, mix again to blend.
9. Mix the bacon and burger back in, let sit for a couple of minutes to warm tenderly back up.
10. Serve

Nutrition Information: Calories 607g, Fat 47g, Carbs 10g, Sugars 4g, Protein 33g

★★ WW INSTANT POT FISH AND SEAFOOD

Easiest Ever Low Carb High Protein Shrimp with Coconut Milk

Prep Time: 10mins, Cook Time: 10mins, Serving: 6, Point value: 8

Ingredients

- 1 - pound shrimp shelled
- 1 - tablespoon minced ginger minced
- 1 - tablespoon garlic minced
- ½ - teaspoon turmeric
- 1 - teaspoon salt
- ½ - teaspoon cayenne pepper
- 1 - teaspoon garam masala
- ½ - can unsweetened coconut milk

Instructions

1. Combine all fixings.
2. In the internal liner of your Instant Pot, place some water, and spot a trivet on top.
3. Spot the shrimp and coconut blend in a pot that fits inside your Instant Pot, and spread with foil.
4. Set your Instant Pot at 4 minutes for low weight, discharge weight rapidly and blend well. Include some additional coconut milk on the off chance that you need.

Nutrition Information: Calories 192g, Fat 12g, Carbs 4g, Sugar 1g, Protein 16g

Instant Pot Indian Fish Curry

Prep Time: 5mins, Cook Time: 10mins, Servings: 4, Point value: 8

Ingredients

- 2 - Tbsp coconut oil
- 10 - curry leaves optional
- 1 - cup onion chopped
- 1 - Tbsp garlic
- 1 - Tbsp ginger
- ½ - jalapeno chili pepper
- 1 - cup tomato chopped
- 1 - tsp ground coriander
- ¼ - tsp ground cumin
- ½ - tsp turmeric
- ½ - tsp black pepper
- 1 - tsp salt
- 2 - Tbsp water for deglazing
- 1 - cup canned coconut milk

- 1 ½ - lbs fish fillets
- 1 tsp lime juice
- Fresh cilantro leaves
- Fresh tomato slices

Instructions

1. Select the 'Saute' work and pre-heat the Instant Pot.
2. Add coconut oil to the pre-warmed inward pot of Instant Pot and permit it to warm up.
3. Include onions, garlic, ginger and green chilies to the inward pot.
4. Blend onion blend until onions are translucent.
5. Include tomatoes and saute until the tomatoes discharge their fluid and start isolating.
6. Include coriander, cumin, turmeric, dark pepper, and salt.
7. Saute until flavors are fragrant, round 30 seconds. Be conscious so as not to devour
8. Cautiously consist of fish pieces.
9. Tenderly raise up the fish portions so the coconut milk achieves the ground of the internal pot, and the fish is protected with the sauce.
10. Close the duvet and weight cook dinner for two minutes.
11. Complete a Quick Release of weight and open the quilt.
12. Tenderly paintings the curry without isolating the fish.
13. Cautiously evacuate fish and sauce right into a serving bowl.
14. Embellishment with hacked cilantro and crisp tomato cuts. Serve over rice.

Nutrition Information: Calories 190g, Fat 11g, Carbs 6g, Sugar 3g, Protein 16g

Brussels Sprouts in the Instant Pot

Prep Time: 10mins, Cooking Time: 10mins, Serving: 4, Point value: 11

Ingredients

- 1 - lb. Brussels Sprouts, Olive Oil, Salt & Pepper, ¼ - C. Pine Nuts

Instructions

1. In the Instant Pot, set the trivet, and after that vicinity the steamer bushel on.
2. Pour in 1 C. Water.
3. By then encompass the Brussels sprouts apex of the steamer field.
4. Lock the apex, and set on Manual for 3mins.
5. At the point whilst the pot is executed (booms) general a brief launch.
6. Season with Olive Oil, Salt, and Pepper, and sprinkle with Pine Nuts.

Nutrition Information: Calories 343g, Fat 8g, Carbs 14g, Sugars 0.4g, Protein 15g

Instant Pot Bone Broth

Prep Time: 10mins, Cook Time: 2hrs 10mins, Serving: 8, Point value: 9

Ingredients

- 1-2 - chicken feet, 1-2 - large carrots, 1 - medium onion
- 2-3 - stalks of celery, 1 - head of garlic smashed
- 1-2 - TB apple cider vinegar & Water enough to cover the bones

Instructions

1. Put the bones into the pot initially pursued with the aid of the veggies, garlic, and apple juice vinegar. Fill the pot with water to cover the bones - ensure you do not go over the "Maximum" line on the pot.
2. Give the pot a risk to sit down for around 30 minutes with no warm temperature to permit the apple juice vinegar to pull the minerals from the bones.
3. Put the Instant Pot cover on and turn the vent valve to shut. Push "Soup" and make use of the guide trap to convey the time so long as a 120mins.
4. The pot will flip "On" certainly and could take around 20 minutes to return to weight before the 120mins start checking down.
5. After 120 minutes of weight cooking is carried out, flip the Instant Pot off and abandon or not it's to commonly discharge around 15mins earlier than beginning the vents valve and stressing your soup.

Nutrition Information: Calories 265g, Fat 11g, Carbs 15g, Sugars 3.2g, Protein 28g

Creamy Shrimp Scampi

Prep Time: 5mins, Cook Time: 10mins, Serving: 4, Point value: 10

Ingredients

- 2 - tablespoons butter
- 1 - pound shrimp, frozen
- 4 - cloves garlic, minced
- ¼ - ½ teaspoons red pepper flakes
- ½ - teaspoons paprika
- 2 - cups Carbanada low carb pasta
- 1 - cup water or chicken broth
- ½ - cup half and half
- ½ - cup parmesan cheese
- salt to taste, pepper

Instructions

1. Liquefy the spread in the Instant Pot or pot.
2. Include garlic and red pepper chips and cook until the garlic is marginally caramelized 1-2 minutes.
3. Include the paprika and afterward the solidified shrimp, salt, pepper, and noodles.
4. Pour in the stock. In the case of utilizing soup, don't include salt above.
5. Cook under strain for 2 minutes a utilization speedy discharge.
6. Turn the pot to Sauté, include cream and cheddar, and mix until softened.

Nutrition Information: Calories 312g, Fat 9g, Carbs 29g, Sugar 1g, Protein 24g

Instant Pot Seafood Gumbo

Prep Time: 10mins, Cooking Time: 15mins, Servings: 8, Point value: 11

Ingredients

- 24 - ounces sea bass filets patted
- 3 - tablespoons ghee
- 3 - tablespoons cajun seasoning or creole seasoning
- 2 - yellow onions diced
- 2 - bell peppers diced
- 4 - celery ribs diced
- 28 - ounces diced tomatoes
- ¼ - cup tomato paste
- 3 - bay leaves
- 1 ½ - cups bone broth
- 2 - pounds medium to large raw shrimp deveined
- Sea salt to taste
- black pepper to taste

Instructions

1. Season the barramundi with a few salt and pepper, and make certain they're as similarly covered as can be predicted under the instances. Sprinkle half of of the Cajun flavoring onto the fish and provide it a blend make certain it's miles
2. Put the ghee within the Instant Pot and push "Sauté". Hold up until it peruses "Hot" and includes the barramundi pieces. Sauté for approximately 4mins, till it looks cooked on the two facets.
3. Include the onions, pepper, celery and then the rest of the Cajun flavoring to the pot and sauté for 2mins until aromatic. Push "Keep Warm/Cancel". Include the cooked fish, diced tomatoes, tomato glue, narrows leaves, and bone stock to the pot and deliver it a nice combination. Set the top lower back at the pot and set it to "Fixing." Push "Manual" and set the correct opportunity for only five minutes
4. When the 5 minutes have finished, push the "Keep warm/Cancel" capture. Warily change the "Fixing" valve over to "Venting," if you want to bodily discharge the majority of the weight. When the weight has been discharged, evacuate the pinnacle and change the placing to "Sauté" another time. Include the shrimp and prepare dinner for around three-4 minutes, or until the shrimp have grew to become out to be hazy.

Nutrition Information: Calories 292g, Fat 18g, Carbs 10g, Sugar 3g, Protein 28g

Instant Pot Brazilian Fish Stew

Ingredients

- 1 - onion
- 1 - red bell pepper
- 5 - cloves garlic
- 14 -ounces canned crushed tomatoes
- 8 - ounces seafood or fish broth
- 6 - ounces canned full-fat coconut milk
- 2 - tablespoons coconut oil
- 1 - tablespoon ground cumin
- 1 - tablespoon smoked paprika
- 1 - teaspoon salt
- ½ - teaspoon black pepper
- ¼ to ½ - teaspoon ground cayenne

For Finishing:

- 1 ½ - pounds firm white fish like cod
- 2 - tablespoons coconut oil
- 1 - tablespoon lime juice
- 1 - tablespoon chopped fresh cilantro

Instructions

1. Add all stew base fixings to the weight cooker pot, and mix until well-blended.
2. Secure and seal the cover. Cook for 10 minutes at a high weight, trailed by a 10-minute regular discharge. Physically discharge remaining weight.
3. Reveal and turn on the saute mode on the weight cooker for medium warmth.
4. Give the stew a chance to bubble for 10 minutes to thicken the sauce, mixing oftentimes. While trusting that the stew will thicken, continue to the following stage to set up the fish.
5. Expel any skin and bones from the fish, and pat dry with paper towels if clammy. Cut into 1-inch pieces.
6. At the point when the stew has thickened, blend in fish until cooked through, around 5 minutes.
7. Mood killer the saute mode. Blend in coconut oil and lime juice until consolidated. Serve in dishes, and top with slashed cilantro or parsley.

Nutrition Information: Calories 320g, Fat 18g, Carb 10g, Sugars 5.5g, Protein 27g

Creamy Shrimp Scampi

Prep Time: 5mins, Cook Time: 10mins, Servings: 4, Point value: 23

Ingredients

- 2 - tablespoons Butter
- 1 - pound shrimp, frozen
- 4 - cloves Garlic
- ¼ - ½ teaspoons Red Pepper Flakes
- ½ - teaspoons Smoked Paprika
- 2 - cups Carbanada low carb pasta
- 1 - cup water or chicken broth
- ½ - cup half and half
- ½ - cup Parmesan Cheese
- Salt to taste
- Ground Black Pepper to taste

Instructions

1. Dissolve the spread in the Instant Pot or pot.
2. Include garlic and red pepper pieces and cook until the garlic is marginally seared 1-2 minutes.
3. Include the paprika and afterward the solidified shrimp, salt, pepper, and noodles.
4. Pour in the soup. In the case of utilizing soup, don't include salt above.
5. Cook under strain for 2 minutes a utilization fast discharge.
6. Turn the pot to Sauté, include cream and cheddar, and mix until softened.

Nutrition Information: Calories 312g, Fat 9g, Carbs 29g, Sugar 1g, Protein 24g

Instant Pot Salmon With Chili-Lime Sauce

Prep Time: 10mins, Cook Time: 5mins, Servings: 2, Point value:

Ingredients

For steaming salmon:

- 2 - salmon fillets
- 1 - cup water
- sea salt to taste
- freshly ground black pepper

For chili-lime sauce:

- 1 - jalapeno seeds
- 1 - lime juiced
- 2 - cloves garlic minced
- 1 - tablespoon honey
- 1 - tablespoon olive oil
- 1 - tablespoon hot water

- 1 - tsp chopped fresh parsley
- ½ - teaspoon paprika
- ½ - teaspoon cumin

Instructions

1. Consolidate and blend all sauce fixings in a bowl with a pourable lip. Put apart.
2. Add water to the load cooker. Spot salmon filets over a steam rack inside the pot.
3. Season the best point of the salmon filets with salt and pepper exactly as you would prefer.
4. Spread and lock the cover. Select the steam mode and trade the cooking time to 5mins at high weight.
5. At the factor whilst the weight cooker is executed, make use of the fast discharge take care of to discharge steam weight and to stop the cooking.
6. Open the top and alternate the salmon to a serving plate. Sprinkle with bean stew lime sauce and serve.

Nutrition Information: Calories 400g, Fat 25g, Carb 10.5g, Sugars 9g, Protein 29g

Keto Instant Pot Clam Chowder

Prep Time: 10mins, Cook Time: 10mins, Servings: 6, Point value: 12

Ingredients

- 8 –ounces nitrate-free bacon
- 1 –quart chicken bone broth
- 2 –pounds frozen cauliflower
- 4 –cloves garlic
- 1- ½ -cups diced onion
- 4 - to 5cupsceleriac root
- 1 –tsp salt or more to taste
- 1 –tsp whole dried thyme
- 1 –tsp black pepper
- ¼ -tsp cayenne pepper
- 16 –ounces bottled juice
- 46.5 - ounce cans clams

Instructions

1. Shakers the onions, and strip and bones the celeriac.
2. Press the Sauté seize. Include cleaved bacon and cook until practically fresh, five to 7 mins. Exchange to a paper towel-lined plate to dissipate.
3. Consist of the bone stock and 2 pounds of solidified cauliflower to the Instant Pot.
4. Spread, lock the pinnacle installation and seal the vent.
5. Press Manual and weight prepare dinner on high for 3 minutes. When it signals, physically discharge the load.
6. Utilizing an opened spoon, change the cooked cauliflower along the garlic to a fast blender or nourishment processor.

7. Heartbeat or mix until absolutely smooth. Put aside.
8. Include the diced onion and celeriac, salt, thyme, pepper, cayenne, and shellfish juice to the juices in the pot.
9. Spread, lock the pinnacle and seal the vent.
10. Press Manual and modify the possibility to 5mins. When it alerts, bodily discharge weight.
11. Include the cooked bacon, the cauliflower "cream", and slashed shellfishes which have been washed in a nice work sifter. Mix the entirety collectively.
12. Taste and adjust seasonings, if fundamental. Serve and admire

Nutrition Information: Calories 283.2g, Fat 19.8g, Carbs 7.1g, Sugars 1.6g, Protein 20.3g

Steamed Shrimp and Asparagus Instant Pot

Prep Time: 35mins, Cooking Time: 48mins, Serving: 4, Point value: 31

Ingredients

- 1 - pound peeled and deveined shrimp
- 1 - bunch of asparagus
- 1 - teaspoon olive oil
- ½ - tablespoon Cajun seasoning

Instructions

1. Add some water to your Instant Pot.
2. Supplement the treated steel steam rack that accompanies your Instant Pot to the base of the pot with the handles up.
3. Spot the asparagus on the steam rack in a solitary layer (or silicone steamer) to go about as a bed for your shrimp.
4. Spot the shrimp over the asparagus.
5. Sprinkle the olive oil on the shrimp and afterward season with the Cajun flavoring.
6. Spread and lock the top.
7. Select "Steam" mode and press the "- " catch until it peruses 2 minutes and after that select "Low Pressure". Additionally, make a point to set the top handle to "Fixing" and not "Venting". I utilized solidified shrimp so you'll need to diminish the opportunity to 1 minute for new shrimp.
8. The Instant Pot will signal at you when it wraps up the shrimp.
9. To maintain a strategic distance from over-cooking, move the top handle from "Fixing" to "Venting" to physically discharge the weight. When the majority of the weight discharges the steam will never again leave the vent and you'll have the option to open the top.

Nutrition Information: Calories 624g, Fat 84g, Carbs 94.5g, Sugar 8.2g, Protein 123g

Instant Pot Bacon Brussels Sprouts recipe

Prep Time: 5mins, Cook Time: 5mins, Serving: 4, Point value: 9

Ingredients

- 16 - oz. fresh Brussels sprouts
- 1 - tablespoon olive oil
- 2 - teaspoons minced garlic
- ½ - white onion chopped
- 6 - slices of bacon chopped
- ½ - teaspoon salt
- ¼ - teaspoon black pepper

Instructions

1. Trim finishes of washed Brussels grows. Cut each down the middle.
2. Add water to your Instant Pot embed. Spot steamer bin inside. Organize Brussels grows in the bushel.
3. Close the IP cover, set valve to fixing, press "manual" or "weight cooking" setting and set the clock to 3 minutes. The weight cooker will take a couple of minutes to come to weight and will begin cooking.
4. When done, rapidly discharge weight by changing the valve to "venting" position.
5. Expel Brussels grows from the Instant Pot. Channel water out of the addition. Set the IP to "sauté" setting. Add olive oil to embed. Include onions and garlic and sauté for 2 minutes. Include bacon and cook until firm and sautéed. Include Brussels sprouts and blend, sautéing for a couple of minutes. Mood killer the IP. Expel Brussels grows onto serving dish.

Nutrition Information: Calories 194g, Fat 13g, Carbs 12g, Sugars 3g, Protein 8g

Instant Pot Steamed Wild-Caught Crab Legs

Prep Time: 15mins, Cook Time: 3mins, Servings: 4, Point value: 12

Ingredients

- 2 – Pounds wild-caught Snow Crab legs, 1 –cup water
- 1/3 -cup salted grass-fed butter, lemon slices

Instructions

1. Spot the metal trivet in the base of your Instant Pot.
2. Include 1 container water.
3. Add the crab legs to the pot. In the event that it defrosts them marginally so you can fit them all in the Instant Pot, that is fine.
4. Spot the cover on the Instant Pot and seal the vent.
5. Press the "Manual" catch and modify the opportunity to 3 minutes.
6. Fast discharge the weight when the Instant Pot signals.
7. Use tongs to painstakingly exchange the cooked crab legs to a platter for serving.

8. Present with dissolved grass-nourished spread and lemon cuts

Nutrition Information: Calories 326g, Fat 11g, Carbs 18g, Sugar 3.4g, Protein 28g

Instant Pot Lemon-Dill Salmon & Asparagus

Prep Time: 10mins, Cook Time: 10mins, Serving: 1, Point value: 17

Ingredients

- 1 - cup pure water
- 3 to 5 large sprigs fresh herbs
- 1 - clove garlic fresh, crushed
- 1 - pound wild-caught Alaskan salmon filet skin-on
- 1 - tsp grass-fed butter ghee
- 1 - teaspoon sea salt
- 1 - teaspoon garlic powder
- ½ - teaspoon dried dill
- 6 to 7 organic lemon

Instructions

1. Include water, new dill, and squashed garlic to the burden cooker embed pot.
2. At that factor place trivet inside as well, with the handles up.
3. Spot salmon, pores and skin side down, over the trivet.
4. In the event that utilizing spread or ghee, speck 1 tablespoon of the fat to the very best point of the salmon.
5. Sprinkle filet with three/four teaspoon ocean salt, garlic granules, and dried dill.
6. Top with lemon cuts in a uniform layer.
7. Spread the pot, checking the seal and parts to make sure the whole lot is brilliant.
8. When making use of an electric powered cooker, set to high weight for 4mins.
9. At the factor when the cycle is completed, divert off or expel from warmth. Fast discharge weight.
10. Expel the cooker cowl, at that point in all respects cautiously, utilizing broiler gloves, expel the trivet from the pot.
11. On the off risk that you want a crispier salmon pinnacle, don't hesitate to put the pieces below a warm grill for round 1 to 2mins.
12. Watch out for it so it doesn't devour!
13. Cautiously raise the pot out of the cooker.
14. Return the supplement pot to cooker. Include final 2 tablespoons of fat.
15. In the event that using an electric powered cooker, for instance, the Instant Pot, press the "Saute" paintings.
16. On the off chance that utilizing a stovetop cooker, location on burner over medium warm temperature.
17. When the fat has dissolved, inclusive of asparagus. Mix incidentally for round 4 to 5mins till desired doneness.
18. Season with amazing 1/4 teaspoon ocean salt.

19. Serve speedy, with asparagus as an afterthought. Embellishment with more lemon cuts, crisp herbs, shaved crude Parmesan, escapades.

Nutrition Information: Calories 343g, Fat 20g, Carbs 88g, Sugars 32g, Protein 76g

Perfectly Steamed Wild-Caught Crab Legs Instant Pot

Cook Time: 3mins, Total Time: 3mins, Servings: 4, Point value: 54

Ingredients

- 2 -pounds wild-caught Snow Crab legs, 1 -cup water
- 1/3 – cup salted grass-fed butter, lemon slices

Instructions

1. Spot the metal trivet in the base of your Instant Pot.
2. Include 1 glass water.
3. Add the crab legs to the pot. On the off chance that it defrosts them somewhat so you can fit them all in the Instant Pot, that is fine.
4. Spot the top on the Instant Pot and seal the vent.
5. Press the "Manual" catch and alter the opportunity to 3 minutes.
6. Snappy discharge the weight when the Instant Pot blares.
7. Use tongs to deliberately exchange the cooked crab legs to a platter for serving.
8. Present with softened grass-nourished spread and lemon cuts

Nutrition Information: Calories 1320g, Fat 52g, Carbs 200g, Sugars 28g, Protein 44g

Instant Pot Lemon Pepper Salmon

Prep Time: 5mins, Cook Time: 10mins, Servings: 3 – 4, Point value: 9

Ingredients

- ¾ - cup water, 1 - pound salmon filet skin on
- 3 - teaspoons ghee or other healthy fat
- ¼ - teaspoon salt or to taste, ½ - teaspoon pepper
- ½ - lemon thinly, 1 - zucchini julienned
- 1 - red bell pepper julienned, 1 - carrot julienned

Instructions

1. Spot salmon, skin down at the rack.
2. Shower salmon with ghee/fats, season with salt and pepper and spread with lemon cuts.
3. Close the Instant Pot and make certain the vent is swung to "Fixing".
4. While salmon chefs, julienne your vegetables.
5. Press the "Warm/Cancel" trap. Evacuate pinnacle, and making use of warm cushions, cautiously expel rack with salmon and set on a plate.
6. Expel herbs and cast off. Include vegetables and set the cover returned on.

7. Press "Sauté" and allow the greens to cook dinner for the simplest 1 or 2 minutes.
8. Serve veggies with salmon and add the last teaspoon of fat to the pot and pour a tad little bit of the sauce over them each time wanted.

Nutrition Information: Calories 296g, Fat 15g, Carbs 8g, Sugar 4g, Protein 31g

Instant Pot Seafood Gumbo

Prep Time: 10mins, Cooking Time: 10mins, Servings: 8, Point value: 6

Ingredients

- 24 - ounces sea bass filets patted dry
- 3 - tablespoons ghee or avocado oil
- 3 - tablespoons cajun seasoning
- 2 - yellow onions
- 2 - bell peppers
- 4 - celery ribs
- 28 - ounces diced tomatoes
- ¼ - cup tomato paste
- 3 - bay leaves
- 1 ½ - cups bone broth
- 2 - pounds medium to large raw shrimp
- sea salt to taste
- black pepper

Instructions

1. Sprinkle 1/2 of the Cajun flavoring onto the fish and provide it a mix make sure it's miles protected properly and placed aside.
2. Put the ghee within the Instant Pot and push "Sauté". Hold up until it peruses "Hot" and includes the barramundi lumps.
3. Sauté for around 4 minutes, until it appears cooked on the 2 facets. Utilize an opened spoon to trade the fish to a large plate.
4. Include the onions, pepper, celery and the remainder of the Cajun flavoring to the pot and sauté for two minutes until fragrant.
5. Include the cooked fish, diced tomatoes, tomato glue, immediately leaves, and bone juices to the pot and supply it a pleasing combo.
6. When the five minutes have finished, push the "Keep heat/Cancel" trap.
7. Circumspectly alternate the "Fixing" valve over to "Venting," on the way to bodily discharge most people of the burden.
8. When the weight has been discharging, evacuate the duvet and exchange the putting to "Sauté" over again.
9. Include the shrimp and cook for around three-four minutes, or until the shrimp have grown to become out to be difficult to understand.
10. Include a few extra ocean salt and dark pepper, to flavor. Serve warm and finish off with a few cauliflower rice and chives.

Nutrition Information: Calories 432g, Fat 19g, Carbs 15g, Sugar 5g, Protein 43g

Instant Pot Brussels Sprouts Gratin

Prep Time: 5mins, Cook Time: 20mins, Serving: 5, Point value: 11

Ingredients

- 16 -oz Whole Brussels Sprouts
- ¾ - cup grated sharp cheddar
- 1 - tablespoon all purpose flour
- 1 - teaspoon fresh thyme leaves
- 1 - clove garlic, peeled and minced fine
- sea salt and cracked pepper
- 1 - cup heavy cream
- ½ - cup pank breadcrumbs
- ½ - cup grated parmesan
- 1 to 2 tablespoons of EVOO

Instructions

1. In a blender, include brussels grows and throb. You don't need them puréed, simply decent and minced. Add to a bowl. Include the Cheddar, flour, thyme, garlic, and some salt and pepper to the bowl. Hurl to join. Add the blend to a 7 Cup Pyrex Dish, pressing it in. Pour over the overwhelming cream.
2. Empty 2 containers warm water into the base of IP liner. A spot in your trivet, and after that place in your pyrex bowl of fixings. Spot a bit of foil over your pyrex bowl. This prevents dampness from getting into it.
3. Spot cover on, and turn onto High Manual Pressure for 14 minutes.
4. Preheat stove to 425 degrees F. When IP is done, complete a QR. You can either utilize a similar pyrex bowl to heat in or empty substance into another broiler safe dish and spread around.
5. In a little bowl, join the panko, Parmesan, and oil and pour over the Brussels grows blend.
6. Prepare until the top is delightful brilliant darker shading. When expelled from broiler, grind some new parmesan on top! Who doesn't love cheddar?

Nutrition Information: Calories 324g, Fat 12g, Carbs 6g, Sugar 2.4g, Protein 22g

High Protein Shrimp with Coconut Milk

Prep Time: 10mins, Cook Time: 10mins, Servings: 5, Point value: 11

Ingredients

- 1 - pound shrimp shelled
- 1 - tablespoon minced ginger
- 1 - tablespoon Garlic

- ½ - teaspoon Turmeric
- 1 - teaspoon Salt
- ½ - teaspoon Cayenne
- 1 - teaspoon Garam Masala
- ½ - can Full-Fat Coconut Milk

Instructions

1. In the inward liner of your Instant Pot, place some water, and spot a trivet on top.
2. Spot the shrimp and coconut blend in a pot that fits inside your Instant Pot, and spread with foil.
3. Set your Instant Pot at 4 minutes for low weight, discharge weight rapidly and blend well. Include some additional coconut milk on the off chance that you need.

Nutrition Information: Calories 192g, Fat 12g, Carbs 4g, Sugar 1g, Protein 16g

Creamy Shrimp Scampi

Prep Time: 5mins, Cook Time: 10mins, Serving: 3, Point value: 10

Ingredients

- 2 - tablespoons butter
- 1 - pound shrimp, frozen
- 4 - cloves garlic, minced
- ¼ - ½ - teaspoons red pepper flakes
- ½ - teaspoons paprika
- 2 - cups Carbanada low carb pasta (uncooked)
- 1 - cup water or chicken broth
- ½ - cup half and half
- ½ - cup parmesan cheese
- salt, to taste
- pepper, to taste

Instructions

1. Dissolve the spread in the Instant Pot or pan.
2. Include garlic and red pepper pieces and cook until the garlic is marginally seared 1-2 minutes.
3. Include the paprika and afterward the solidified shrimp, salt, pepper, and noodles.
4. Pour in the soup. In the case of utilizing stock, don't include salt above.
5. Cook under strain for 2 minutes a utilization fast discharge.
6. Turn the pot to Sauté, include cream and cheddar, and blend until dissolved.

Nutrition Information: Calories 312g, Fat 9g, Carbs 29g, Sugar 1g, Protein 24g

★★ WW INSTANT POT POULTRY

Fall-Off-The-Bone Chicken

Prep Time: 10mins, Cook Time: 35mins, Serves: 10, Point value: 10

Ingredients

- 1 - whole - 4lb. organic chicken
- 1 - Tbsp. Organic Virgin Coconut Oil
- 1 - tsp. paprika
- 1½ - cups Pacific Organic Bone Broth Chicken
- 1 - tsp. dried thyme
- ¼ - tsp. freshly ground black pepper
- 2 - Tbsp. lemon juice, ½ - tsp. sea salt, 6 - cloves garlic

Instructions

1. In a little bowl, consolidate paprika, thyme, salt, and pepper. Rub flavoring over outside of winged creature.
2. Warmth oil in the weight cooker to gleaming. Include chicken, bosom side down and cook 6-7 minutes.
3. Flip the chicken and include stock, lemon juice, and garlic cloves.
4. Lock weight cooker top and set for 25 minutes on high.
5. Give the weight cooker a chance to discharge normally.
6. Expel from weight cooker and let represent 5 minutes before cutting.

Nutrition Information: Calories: 235g, Fat 22g, Carbs 12g, Sugar 4g, Protein 35g

Yummy Shredded Chicken

Prep Time: 20mins, Cooking Time: 30mins, Serving: 1, Point value: 5

Ingredients

- 4 - lbs chicken breasts or 18 chicken tenders
- ½ - c water or chicken broth, 1 - tsp salt, ½ - tsp pepper

Instructions

1. Include most of the fixings to the Instant Pot.
2. Press the "chicken" trap at that factor utilizing the likewise to picture comprise of five minutes for a blend of 20 minutes.
3. If you are using cemented meat, include an extra 5mins for tenders and 10 minutes for chests.
4. At the point when the weight cooking time has finished, cautiously redirect the valve from "fixing" to "vent" to fast weight release.
5. Recognize the fowl onto a plate or cutting board and permit it cool for a few minutes.
6. Use forks to shred.

7. Store the hen in an impermeable compartment with a piece of the liquid to help keep up the meat sticky.

Nutrition Information: Calories 200.2g, Fat 5.2g, Carbs 7.1g, Sugars 0.6g, Protein 29.3g

Instant Pot Buffalo Chicken Meatballs

Prep Time: 10mins, Cook Time: 20mins, Servings: 6, Point value: 16

Ingredients

- 1.5 - lb ground chicken
- ¾ - cup almond meal
- 1 - tsp sea salt
- 2 - garlic cloves minced
- 2 - green onions thinly
- 2 - tbsp ghee
- 6 - tbsp hot sauce
- 4 - tbsp ghee or butter
- Chopped green onions

Instructions

1. In an extensive bowl, join chicken, almond supper, salt, minced garlic cloves, and green onions.
2. Utilize your hands to consolidate everything together, except be mindful so as not to exhaust the meat.
3. Oil your hands with ghee or coconut oil, at that point shape the meat into balls 1-2 inches wide.
4. While the meatballs are searing, consolidate hot sauce and 4 tbsp of spread or ghee and warmeth them in the microwave or the stove top until the margarine is totally liquefied. Utilize a spoon to mix. This is your wild ox sauce.
5. Spot all the sautéed meatballs in the Instant Pot, at that point pour the wild ox sauce equitably over the meatballs.
6. Screw on the top to the Instant Pot, ensure that the weight valve is set to "fixing," at that point set it to "Poultry."
7. When the meatballs are done cooking, the Instant Pot will signal. In the event that you are consuming right, hit "Drop" at that point discharge the weight valve, ensuring your hand is far from the opening where the steam get away. If not, the Instant Pot will naturally change to the "Warm" setting for the following 10 hours and the weight will gradually bring down without anyone else.
8. Serve over rice, cauliflower rice, zoodles. or then again simply eat without anyone else!

Nutrition Information: Calories 357g, Fat 28g, Carbs 3g, Sugar 1.2g, Protein 23g

Pressure Cooker Chicken Puttanesca

Prep Time: 10mins, Cook Time: 15mins, Servings: 6, Point value: 19

Ingredients

- 6 - chicken thighs
- 2 - tablespoons extra virgin olive oil
- 2 - cloves garlic
- salt and freshly milled black pepper
- ½ - tsp red chilli flakes
- 14 ½ - oz canned chopped tomatoes
- 6 - oz pitted black olives
- 1 - tbsp capers , rinsed and drained
- 1 - tbsp chopped fresh basil
- ¾ - cup water

Instructions

1. Turn on the 'sauté' work in your Instant Pot or other electric powered weight cooker and encompass the oil. Hold up 1 minute and include the bird portions skin side down, numerous pieces at any given second till they may be seared and in no way again adhere to the bottom of the pot, around five minutes or somewhere within the region.
2. With the sauté potential still on, include the cleaved tomatoes, water, olives, garlic, escapades, hacked basil, crimson bean stew chips, and a few salt and pepper.
3. Blend the whole thing extraordinary, bring it up to a sensitive stew, at that point supplant the chook thighs within the pot.
4. Turn to sauté capacity off.
5. Lock the top, flip the vent to 'fixing' and utilizing the manual setting, and alter it to cook dinner for 15mins at High Pressure.
6. At the point when the cooking time is up, allow the unit to lessen weight alone without establishing the steam discharge vent for at any charge 12 minutes.
7. Following 12 minutes you could carefully and step by step discharge the rest of the weight.
8. Present with an aspect of vegetables, I applied zucchini noodles.

Nutrition Information: Calories 343g, Fat 27g, Carbs 4g, Sugars 1g, Protein 19g

Instant Pot Spaghetti Squash Chicken Alfredo

Prep Time: 5mins, Cook Time: 35mins, Serving: 5, Point value: 19

Ingredients

- 1 - Whole spaghetti squash
- 16 - oz skinless chicken breasts
- 4 – oz. cream cheese softened
- ½ - cup low-sodium chicken broth

- 2 - cups broccoli chopped
- 1 - cup parmesan cheese
- ¼ - cup heavy whipping cream
- ¾ - tbsp butter softened
- 1 - tbsp flour
- 1 - tbsp minced garlic
- 2 - cups almond milk
- 1 - cup water
- 1 - tsp olive oil

Instructions

1. Cut the spaghetti squash down the middle, across. Scoop out the seeds and dispose of.
2. Add some water to the pot. Spot the spaghetti squash parts in the moment pot, with the cut sides looking up.
3. Spot the cover on the weight cooker and cook on high weight for 7 minutes.
4. After the 7 minutes, fast discharge the valve at the highest point of the weight cooker to bring down the weight.
5. Evacuate the top and the squash. Jab the squash to guarantee it's delicate. Shred the squash with a fork to make "spaghetti."
6. Spill out the abundance of water from the Instant Pot.
7. Season the chicken bosom blocks with the seasonings.
8. Add the olive oil to the pot. At the point when the oil is warm include the chicken.
9. Saute' the two sides of the chicken until darker and cooked.
10. Include the minced garlic and cook until fragrant. Deglaze the pot by including the chicken juices.
11. Include the almond milk, whipping cream, cream cheddar, and margarine to the pot.
12. Add the chicken back to the pot. Blend well to join.
13. Add extra salt and pepper to taste if necessary.
14. Serve the chicken and cream sauce over the spaghetti squash.

Nutrition information: calories 368.1g, fat 32.1g, carbs 5.3g, sugars 3.3g, protein 15.9g

Chicken Chili Instant Pot No Beans

Prep Time: 20mins, Cook Time: 30mins, Serving: 8, Point value: 6

Ingredients

- 1 ½ - pounds frozen chicken breast
- 8 - ounces cream cheese
- ½ - teaspoon cumin
- 2 - teaspoons salt
- 20 - ounces chicken broth
- ½ - teaspoon chili powder
- ½ - teaspoon pepper

- 10 - oz diced tomatoes with green chilies
- Shredded Mexican cheese
- Avocado
- Sour cream

Instructions

1. Spot chicken, solidified into the weight cooker.
2. Include every other fixing aside from whatever is for embellishment, including cream cheddar last.
3. Cook at a high weight for 15 minutes then NPR 15 minutes and QR any extra weight.
4. Expel cover and cautiously evacuate chicken and shred at that point blend all fixings together.
5. Present with any of the above embellishments or any of your top choices.

Nutrition Information: Calories 207g, Fat 5g, Carbs 3g, Sugar 1g, Protein 20g

Buffalo Chicken Lettuce Wraps Instant Pot

Prep Time: 5mins, Cooking Time: 4hrs, Serving: 6, Point value: 3

Ingredients
For the chicken:
- 24 – oz boneless skinless chicken breasts
- 1 - celery stalk
- ½ - onion, diced
- 1 - clove garlic
- 16 - oz fat free low sodium chicken broth
- ½ - cup cayenne pepper sauce

For the wraps:
- 6 - large lettuce leaves, Bibb or Iceberg
- 1 ½ - cups shredded carrots
- 2 - large celery stalks, cut into 2 inch matchsticks

Instructions

1. Consolidate chicken, onions, celery stalk, garlic and juices in the Instant Pot. Spread and cook high weight 15 minutes. Normal discharge.
2. Expel the chicken from pot, hold 1/2 glass juices and dispose of the rest. Shred the chicken with two forks, come back to the pot with the 1/2 glass stock and the hot sauce and saute 2 to 3 minutes. Makes 3 containers chicken.
3. To plan lettuce containers, place 1/2 glass bison chicken in each leaf, top with 1/4 glass destroyed carrots, celery, and dressing of your decision. Wrap up and begin eating

Nutrition Information: Calories: 147.5g, Fat 0.1g, Carbs 5.2g, Sugar 1.5g, Protein 25g

Keto Instant Pot Crack Chicken Recipe

Prep time: 5mins, Cook time: 20mins, Serving: 8, Point value: 17

Ingredients

- 2 - slices bacon, chopped
- 910g - boneless, skinless chicken breasts
- 227g - blocks cream cheese
- ½ - cup water
- 2 - tablespoons apple cider vinegar
- 1 - tablespoon dried chives
- 1½ - teaspoons garlic powder
- 1½ - teaspoons onion powder
- 1 - teaspoon crushed red pepper flakes
- 1 - teaspoon dried dill
- ¼ - teaspoon salt
- ¼ - teaspoon black pepper
- 57g - shredded cheddar
- 1 - scallion, green and white parts

Instructions

1. Turn weight cooker on, press "Sauté", and trust that the pot will warm up. Include the hacked bacon and cook until fresh. Exchange to a plate and put aside. Press "Drop" to quit sautéing.
2. Include the chicken, cream cheddar, water, vinegar, chives, garlic powder, onion powder, pounded red pepper pieces, dill, salt, and dark pepper to the pot. Turn the pot on Manual, High Pressure for 15 minutes and after that complete a fast discharge.
3. Use tongs to exchange the chicken to a vast plate, shred it with 2 forks, and return it back to the pot.
4. Blend in the cheddar.
5. Top with the fresh bacon and scallion, and serve.

Nutrition Information: Calories: 437g, Fat 27.6g, Carbs 4.5g, Sugar 2.1g, Protein 41.2

Instant Pot Lemon Chicken with Garlic

Prep Time: 9mins, Cook Time: 20mins, Servings: 1, Point value: 18

Ingredients

- 6-8 - boneless chicken thighs
- sea salt and pepper to taste
- ½ - teaspoon garlic powder
- ½ - teaspoon smoked paprika
- ½ - teaspoon red chili flakes
- 2 - Tablespoons olive oil
- 3 - Tablespoons butter
- ½ - small onion
- 4 - garlic cloves

- Juice of 1 lemon
- 2-4 - teaspoons Italian seasoning
- zest of half a lemon
- 1/3 - cup chicken broth
- 2 - Tablespoons heavy cream

Instructions

1. Press the Sauté work on the Instant Pot and add the olive oil to the pot.
2. Spot chicken in the Instant Pot and cook on each side for 2-3 minutes.
3. When seared, expel from Instant Pot and put aside.
4. Liquefy margarine in Instant Pot and blend in the onions and garlic.
5. Spot the chicken over into the Instant Pot, lock the cover, and turn the valve to fixing.
6. It will take around 5-10 minutes to come to weight and begin tallying down.
7. Discharge the weight for 2mins at that point evacuates your Instant Pot top.
8. Expel chicken from Instant Pot utilizing tongs and put aside on a vast serving plate. Blend in substantial cream into the Instant Pot.
9. On the off chance that you like your sauce thicker, you can thicken with a cornstarch slurry.
10. Cook and enable the sauce to bubble and thicken.
11. Mood killer and add the chicken back to the Instant Pot to coat with sauce. Spoon sauce over chicken and sprinkle with slashed parsley.
12. Present with your preferred sides and embellishment with lemon cuts, whenever wanted.

Nutrition Information: Calories 366g, Fat 31g, Carbs 2g, Sugar 3.1g, Protein 18g

Instant Pot Chicken Wings

Prep Time: 5mins, Cook Time: 22mins, Servings: 6, Point Value: 42

Ingredients

- 5 - lbs. Chicken Wings
- ¼ - C Apple Cider Vinegar
- 1 - Tbsp Cayenne Pepper
- 1 - Tbsp Ghee
- 1 - Tsp Black Pepper
- 1 - Tsp Sea Salt

Extra Sauce for Coating
- ½ - C Hot Sauce
- 3 - Tbsp Ghee

Instructions

1. Join warm sauce, vinegar, cayenne pepper, ghee, dark pepper, ocean salt in a medium and whisk.
2. Save ¼ C of the sauce for seasoning and overlaying later.
3. Expel wing pointers from the primary drummettes, and separate the pads.

4. In the internal pot of the Instant Pot, be part of the chicken wings and sauce.
5. Blend the wings and sauce well together.
6. At the factor when prepared to make the wings, switch on the Instant Pot.
7. Put the liner pot with the hen wings in the pot, near the top and flip the vent valve to "Shut" role.
8. Press "Manual". Press till the clock is going all the way down to 10mins.
9. In the period in-between, activate the broiler to "Sear" and line a treat sheet with cloth paper.
10. At the factor when the clock goes off, allow the presser discharge commonly and open the duvet whilst the vent goes with the flow valve opens.
11. Take out the bird wings, and notice them in a solitary layer at the lined deal with a sheet.
12. Treat the bird wings with the rest of the saved hot sauce.
13. Sear for round 5mins or till cooked, without consuming the skin.
14. In the interim, make the extra sauce for masking and serving.
15. At the factor, while the wings are darkish colored, turn the portions over to sear the other aspect.
16. At the factor, while the wings are performed, take out the wings to a serving platter, sprinkle with extra sauce.
17. Serve fast with carrots and celery sticks.

Nutrition Information: Calories: 939g, Fat 70g, Carbs 1g, Sugar 5.3g, Protein 69g

Belizean Stewed Chicken in the Instant Pot

Prep Time: 15mins, Cooking Time: 15mins, Serving: 3, Point value: 16

Ingredients

- 4 - whole chicken legs
- 1 - Tbsp coconut oil
- 2 - Tbsp recado rojo
- 2 - Tbsp white vinegar
- 3 - Tbsp Worcestershire sauce
- 1 - cup sliced yellow onions
- 3 - cloves garlic
- 1 - tsp ground cumin
- 1 – tsp. dried oregano
- ½ - tsp ground black pepper
- 1 - Tbsp granulated sugar substitute
- 2 - cups chicken stock

Instructions

1. Consolidate the recado or achiote glue, vinegar, Worcestershire sauce, cumin, oregano, pepper and sugar in an expansive bowl.
2. Include the hook portions and rub the marinade into the skin.

3. Marinate for in any event one hour up to medium-term.
4. Spot the supplement for your Instant Pot and set to sauté.
5. Warmth the coconut oil and darkish colored the chook in clumps, skin side down for around 2mins for each facet
6. Expel the blistered fowl to a plate and placed aside.
7. Add the hen pieces returned to the Instant Pot.
8. Empty the chook inventory into the bowl containing the rest of the marinade and mix well.
9. Pour the juices/marinade over the hen pieces within the Instant Pot.
10. Seal the Instant Pot as in step with producer's hints.
11. Set the Instant Pot to Manual, High weight, for 20mins.
12. At the factor when the clock goes off, discharge the steam.
13. Taste the sauce and include really salt if necessary at that factor serve the fowl hot, decorated with cilantro every time wanted.

Nutrition Information: Calories 391g, Fat 22g, Carbs 9g, Sugar 4g, Protein 28g

Instant Pot Chicken Tikka Masala

Prep Time: 5mins, Cook Time: 25mins, Servings: 6, Point value: 9

Ingredients

- 2 - lbs boneless skinless chicken breast
- 1 - small onion
- ½ - yellow bell pepper
- 2 - tablespoons butter
- 1 - teaspoon cumin
- 1 - teaspoon coriander
- 2 - teaspoons garam masala
- 1 - teaspoon turmeric
- ¼ - teaspoon cayenne pepper
- 1 ½ - teaspoon sea salt
- 15 - oz can diced tomatoes
- ½ - cup full fat coconut milk
- 3 - cloves garlic, minced
- 1 - teaspoon grated fresh ginger

Instructions

1. Set your Instant Pot to Saute. Include spread, onion, and yellow peppers and cook for three-four minutes until veggies start to mellow.
2. Include garlic, ginger, flavors, and salt and prepare dinner for a further 1-2 minutes.
3. Include tomatoes and coconut milk and mix well to consolidate. Spot chook over combo.
4. Close the pinnacle and set to Poultry.
5. At the point whilst the cycle is completed, expel hen and shred.
6. Appropriating a submersion hand blender, puree the sauce.
7. Add the chicken returned to the sauce and change flavoring to taste.

Nutrition Information: Calories: 280g, Fat 13g, Carbs 6g, Sugar 2g, Protein 33g

Frozen Chicken in the Instant Pot

Prep Time: 30mins, Cooking Time: 20mins, Servings 6 -8, Point value: 8

Ingredients

- 2 - lbs frozen chicken, ½ - cup water, Salt pepper

Instructions

1. Shower the Instant Pot embed with cooking oil.
2. Spot the chicken in the pot, season liberally with salt and pepper and some other seasonings wanted.
3. Pour 1/2 glass water around the sides of the chicken in the pot.
4. Ensure the fixing ring (inside the top) is in the best possible position.
5. Spot the top on the pot and set to the lock or SEAL position.
6. Turn the Instant Pot to the MANUAL setting for 12 minutes. On the off chance that the chicken isn't solidified, 8 minutes will work.
7. Press the MANUAL catch to begin the cooking procedure.
8. At the point when the clock goes off and the chicken is cooked, the weight might be discharged physically via cautiously turning the valve over the Instant Pot to the VENTING position, or essentially enable the strain to normally discharge for around 10-15 minutes before expelling cover.
9. Expel chicken from the pot, shred or cleave and use as required.

Nutrition Information: Calories 297.8g, Fat 6.5g, Carbs 25.1g, Sugars 2.8g, Protein 32.6g

Instant Pot Chicken Breasts

Prep Time: 2mins, Cook Time: 20mins, Servings: 3, Point value: 7

Ingredients

- 1 - Tablespoon oil
- 3 - boneless, skinless chicken breasts
- ¼ - teaspoon garlic salt per chicken breast
- dash black pepper
- 1/8 - teaspoon dried oregano
- 1/8 - teaspoon dried basil
- 1 - cup water

Instructions

1. Preheat the sauté work on the Instant Pot at the most elevated setting and add oil to the pot.
2. Season one side of the chicken bosoms.

3. After the showcase peruses "hot," cautiously include the chicken bosoms, prepared side down, to the pot. I use tongs to keep away from hot oil splatter.
4. Include flavoring the second side.
5. Cook around 3 to 4 minutes on each side, and expel from the pot with the tongs.
6. Add container water to the pot, in addition to the trivet.
7. Spot the chicken on the trivet.
8. Lock the top, and cook on manual high for 5 minutes.
9. Enable the chicken to normally discharge for 5 minutes and after that snappy discharge the rest.
10. Expel the chicken from the pot, and permit to rest for around 5 minutes before serving for most extreme succulence.

Nutrition Information: Calories 243g, Fat 1g, Carbs 46g, Sugar 3g, Protein 9g

Instant Pot Chicken Cacciatore

Prep Time: 10mins, Cooking Time: 25mins, Serving: 4, Point value: 3

Ingredients

- 4 - chicken thighs
- kosher salt and fresh pepper to taste
- olive oil spray
- 14 – oz. crushed tomatoes
- ½ - cup diced onion
- ¼ - cup diced red bell pepper
- ½ - cup diced green bell pepper
- ½ - teaspoon dried oregano
- 1 - bay leaf
- 2 - tablespoons chopped basil

Instructions

1. Season bird with salt and pepper on every side.
2. Press sauté at the Instant Pot, delicately sprinkle with oil and darkish shaded bird on the 2 viewpoints a few minutes.
3. Sprinkle with unbelievably extra oil and consist of onions and peppers.
4. Sauté until decrease and remarkable, 5 minutes.
5. Pour tomatoes over the fowl and veggies, encompass oregano, gulf leaf, salt, and pepper, deliver it a fast combination and unfurl.
6. Cook high weight 25mins; highlight launch.
7. Oust gulf leaf, upgrade with parsley and serve over pasta, squats or something you need

Nutrition Information: Calories: 133g, Fat 3g, Carbs 10.5g, Sugar 5g, Protein 14g

Bruschetta Chicken

Prep Time: 10mins, Cook Time: 7mins, Servings: 6, Point value: 6

Ingredients

- 2 - lbs chicken breast boneless
- 1 - tbsp olive oil
- ½ - cup chicken broth
- salt and pepper to taste

Tomato Sauce:
- 1 - can diced tomatoes 15 oz
- 1 - tsp oregano
- 4 - cloves garlic
- ¼ - cup balsamic vinegar
- 1 - tsp basil

Instructions

1. Consolidate all factors for the tomato sauce in a bowl. Put apart.
2. Set your Instant Pot to sauté. Give it a risk to take a seat for 2mins and encompass olive oil. Spot four-five bird strips in the pot and allow singeing for 30 seconds. Flip and singe for a further 30 seconds. Exchange to plate and rehash with the staying chicken. Softly season with salt and pepper.
3. Turn the pot to off/keep warm. Tip: I find after I lay the remaining one inside the pot the time has come to turn the primary.
4. Include chicken soup and make use of a wood spoon to deglaze something left at the pot.
5. Include one-portion of the tomato combo and the chicken to the pot.
6. At the point while the pot has got executed with cooking allow a feature discharge for 5mins and after that entire a brisk discharge to evacuate any incredible weight.
7. Expel the fowl and serve over your preferred noodles. Top with the relaxation of the tomato sauce and topped with crispy basil.
8. You can likewise utilize any cooking fluid sauce left inside the Instant Pot but it'll possibly be very moderate.

Nutrition Information: Calories 218g, Fat 6g, Carbs 5g, Sugars 3g, Protein 32g

Instant Pot Faux-tisserie Chicken

Prep Time: 5mins, Cook Time: 33mins, Servings: 4 , Point value 19

Ingredients

- 3 - pound whole chicken
- 2 - Tablespoons olive oil
- sea salt & black pepper
- ½ - medium onion

- 5 - large cloves fresh garlic
- 1 - cup chicken stock/broth

Southwest Seasoning:
- 1 - teaspoon garlic powder
- 1 - teaspoon onion powder
- 1 - teaspoon chili powder
- ½ - teaspoon cumin
- ½ - teaspoon basil

Instructions

1. Spot the onion wedges and garlic cloves inside the chicken. Utilize butcher's twine to verify the legs.
2. Turn on the weight cooker and press the Saute catch.
3. Add the staying olive oil to the metal skillet.
4. Whenever hot, include the chicken and burn/dark colored the two sides, around 4mins
5. Evacuate the chicken and put aside. Spot the trivet at the base of the metal skillet and include the chicken stock.
6. Sprinkle flavoring blend over the whole chicken, scouring it in and spreading it around to cover the whole chicken.
7. Spot the chicken, bosom side up over the trivet and secure the top.
8. Set the weight cooker to Manual and set clock for 25 minutes.
9. At the point when the clock blares, enable the strain to discharge normally for 15mins.
10. In the event that the cover won't open, fast discharge the rest of the weight and evacuate the chicken.
11. Enable chicken to rest for 5 to 10 minutes before serving.

Nutrition Information: Calories: 443g, Fat 32g, Carbs 3g, Sugar 1g, Protein 32g

Paleo Instant Pot Butter Chicken

Prep Time: 5mins, Cook Time: 10mins, Servings: 5, Point value: 10

Ingredients

- 4 - tbsp ghee dairy-free clarified butter
- 10 - garlic cloves
- 1 - tbsp fresh ginger root
- 2- 3 large shallots
- 2 - lbs chicken thighs
- Two 14 oz. diced fire roasted tomatoes
- ¼ - cup full fat coconut milk
- Cilantro, , garnish
- Salt and pepper to taste

Instant Pot Butter Chicken Dry Spice Seasonings:
- 1 - tbsp garam masala powder
- 2 - tsp smoked paprika

- 1.5 - tsp coriander powder
- 2 - tsp turmeric powder

Instructions

1. Generally slash garlic cloves, ginger, and shallots. Join fixings under "Dry Spice Seasonings" in one bowl. Put aside.
2. Moment Pot: Press Sauté capacity - includes 2 tbsp ghee. At the point when the oil is softened, include slashed garlic, ginger, and shallots. Season with a squeeze of salt. Sauté until fragrant. Include Dry Spice Seasonings. Give a brisk sauté to somewhat heat up the flavors. Mood killer Sauté capacity.
3. Include 2 jars of flame cooked tomato and rub the base of the pot to guarantee that nothing adheres to the base.
4. Include chicken and spread the sauce over every piece. Seal the cover and valve. Press Manual - 10 minutes.
5. Whenever done, characteristic discharge until the valve drops.
6. Scoop out the chicken. Include ¼ glass full-fat coconut milk and 2 tbsp ghee. Puree the sauce utilizing a drenching blender until velvety smooth. Dice the chicken to nibble sizes and add them back to the sauce pot. Give it a mix and embellishment with hacked cilantro.
7. Serve the margarine chicken over somewhat cooked cauliflower rice or squashed potatoes.

Nutrition Information: Calories 254g, Fat 15g, Carbs 7g, Sugar 3.5g, Protein 24g

Keto Creamy Chicken Bacon Chowder

Prep Time: 10mins, Cook Time: 30mins, Servings: 4-6, Point value: 20

Ingredients

- 6 - boneless chicken thighs
- 8 - ounce cream cheese full fat
- 4 - t minced garlic
- 1 - C frozen chopped onion celery mix
- 6 - ounce sliced mushrooms
- 4 - T butter
- 1 - t thyme
- salt and pepper to taste

On Cooking Day:
- 3 - C chicken broth
- 1 - C heavy cream
- 1 - pound cooked bacon chopped
- 2 - C fresh spinach

Instructions

To Assemble:

1. 3D shape chicken thighs and add to huge zipper sack.
2. Add remaining fixings to chicken in zipper sack. Speed to seal.

To Cook:

3. Empty chicken blend into Instant Pot, include chicken stock and cook for 30 minutes.
4. Blend well at that point include spinach and cream. Spread and let sit for 10 minutes to shrivel spinach. Top with cleaved bacon.

Nutrition Information: Calories 368.1g, Fat 32.1g, Carbs 5.3g, Sugars 3.3g, Protein 15.9g

Keto Garlic "Butter" Chicken Recipe

Prep Time: 5mins, Cook Time: 40mins, Serving: 4, Point value:

Ingredients

- 4 - chicken breasts
- ¼ - cup turmeric ghee
- 1 - teaspoon salt
- 10 - cloves garlic

Instructions

1. Add the chicken bosoms to the weight cooker pot.
2. Include the ghee, salt, and diced garlic to the weight cooker pot.
3. Set weight cooker on high weight for 35 minutes. Adhere to your weight cooker's directions for discharging the weight.
4. Shred the chicken bosom in the pot.
5. Present with extra ghee if necessary.

Nutrition Information: Calories: 404g, Fat 21g, Carbs 3g, Sugar 0.2g, Protein 47g

★★ WW INSTANT POT BEEF AND PORK

Mississippi Pot Roast

Prep Time: 20mins, Cooking Time: 15mins, Serving: 4-6, Point value: 25

Ingredients

- 3-4 - lb roast
- 1 - packet ranch seasoning mix
- 1 - stick butter
- ½ - jar Peppercorns with the juice
- ½ - cup water

Instructions

1. Spot your dish in the base of your moment pot.
2. Sprinkle the farm blend over the dish.
3. Spot the stick of spread on top and pour the Peppercorns over it.
4. Pour water around the dish.
5. Include the cover and ensure it is swung to fixing. Snap the manual catch and change the opportunity to an hour and a half.
6. Shred and Serve

Nutrition Information: Calories 698g, Fat 39g, Carbs 3g, Sugar 2.4g, Protein 75g

Favorite Instant Pot Taco Meat

Prep Time: 5mins, Cook Time: 10mins, Servings: 8, Point value: 7

Ingredients

- 2 - lbs ground turkey or beef
- ½ - cup finely diced onion
- ½ - cup finely diced bell peppers any color
- 1 - cup unsalted tomato sauce
- 3 - tablespoons homemade taco
- 1 - teaspoon avocado or olive oil
- fresh cilantro

Instructions

1. Utilizing the saute capacity on your Instant Pot, dark colored the meat in the oil. Mood killer saute capacity.
2. Include the rest of the fixings and mix to join. Set pot for 8 minutes on Manual capacity.
3. At the point when the cycle is finished, fast discharge the weight. Brimming with new cilantro whenever wanted.

Nutrition Information: Calories 194g, Fat 10g, Carbs 4g, Sugar 2g, Protein 21g

Keto Beef Brisket in the Instant Pot

Prep Time: 5mins, Cook Time: 66mins, Serving: 8, Point value: 17

Ingredients

- 2.5 - lb beef brisket
- ¼ - cup Keto BBQ seasoning
- 2 - tablespoons avocado
- 4 - slices peeled onion
- 2/3 - cup water
- 2 - tablespoons apple cider vinegar
- 2 - tablespoons low sugar ketchup

Instructions

1. Rub brisket on all sides with bbq flavoring.
2. Warmth oil in Instant Pot on Saute capacity.
3. Spot the prepared brisket into the pot and singe for 3 minutes for every side.
4. Expel with tongs and include the four cuts of onion to the base of the pot.
5. Spot the brisket, fat side up over the onions.
6. Whisk together the water, apple juice vinegar, and ketchup. Pour around the brisket.
7. Spread and seal as per producer's directions.
8. Set to Manual, High Pressure and enter an hour on the clock.
9. At the point when completed the process of cooking, utilize the speedy discharge capacity to expel steam and weight.
10. When all steam is expelled, open and cautiously evacuates the cover.
11. Evacuate the brisket to a cutting board and let it rest for 10 minutes before cutting.
12. Serve the cut brisket with the onions and container juices.

Nutrition Information: Calories 380g, Fat 28g, Carbs 1g, Sugar 0.5g, Protein 29g

Easy Keto Balsamic Beef Pot Roast

Prep Time: 25mins, Cooking Time: 45mins, Serving: 4, Point value: 17

Ingredients

- One boneless chuck roast
- 1 - Tbsp kosher salt
- 1 - tsp black ground pepper
- 1 - tsp garlic powder
- ¼ - cup of balsamic vinegar
- 2 - cups water
- ½ - cup onion
- ¼ - tsp xanthan

- gum
- Fresh parsley

Instructions

1. Cut your toss cook dinner down the middle so you have pieces. Season the dish with the salt, pepper, and garlic powder on all aspects. Utilizing the sauté component on the moment pot, dark colored the meal portions on the two facets.
2. Include a few balsamic vinegar, 1 glass water, and half box onion to the meat. Spread and seal, at that point utilizing the manual catch set the clock for 40mins. At the point while the clock runs out, discharge the load via shifting the transfer to the "venting" setting. When all the weight is discharged, display the pot.
3. Cautiously expel the meat from the skillet to a sizeable bowl. Break cautiously into lumps and evacuate any big bits of fats or other declines.
4. Utilize the sauté capability to warmness the staying fluid to the factor of boiling within the pot, and stew for 10 minutes to lessen.
5. Rush within the thickener, at that point, upload the beef again to the skillet and mix delicately.
6. Mood killer the warmth and serve warm over cauliflower puree, embellished with lots of crisp cleaved parsley.

Nutrition Information: Calories 393g, Fat 28g, Carbs 3g, Sugar 1.5g, Protein 30g

Instant Pot Pulled Pork Recipe

Prep Time: 5mins, Cook Time: 1hr 30mins, Servings: 8, Point value: 6

Ingredients

- 1 - tablespoon chili powder
- 1 - teaspoon coarse sea salt
- 3 - pounds boneless pork shoulder
- 1 ½ - cup Sugar Free BBQ Sauce

Instructions

1. Combine bean stew powder and salt in a little bowl.
2. Cut pork into around 1 lbs pieces. Rub each piece with stew salt blend.
3. Pour half of the BBQ sauce in Instant Pot. Mastermind pork pieces in a solitary layer. Pour remaining sauce over pork.
4. Cook on manual or weight cook at a high weight for an hour and a half. Let weight normally discharge.
5. Take out pork and shred the meat with two forks. Add dish juices to dampen the destroyed pork exactly as you would prefer

Nutrition Information: Calories 247g, Fat 5g, Carbs 4g, Sugar 3g, Protein 38g

Instant Pot Corned Beef and Cabbage

Prep Time: 10mins, Cooking Time: 15mins, Serving: 4, Point value: 28

Ingredients

- 2.5 - lb corned beef
- 1 - head of cabbage
- 4-5 - carrots cut into chunks
- 1 - cup of LOW sodium vegetable broth
- 1 - cup water

Instructions

1. Toss corned hamburger and flavor bundle into the pot with the juices and water. Cook on manual high weight for 85 minutes.
2. At the point when the clock goes off complete a brisk discharge and expel the meat.
3. Include veggies into the juices blend and cook on manual high weight for 4 minutes. At the point when the clock is up to play out a snappy discharge.
4. Present with a side of mustard and appreciate

Nutrition Information: Calories 642g, Fat 42g, Carbs 17g, Sugars 10g, Protein 46g

Instant Pot Beef Bourguignon

Prep Time: 30mins, Cook Time: 50mins, Servings: 6, Point value: 6

Ingredients

- 1.5 - 2 pounds beef roast
- 5 - strips bacon
- 1 - small onion
- 10 -ounces cremini mushrooms quartered
- 2 - carrots chopped
- 5 - cloves garlic
- 3 - bay leaves
- ¾ - cup dry red wine
- ¾ - teaspoon xanthan gum
- 1 - tablespoon tomato paste
- 1 - teaspoon dried thyme
- salt & pepper

Instructions

1. Liberally season meat portions with salt and pepper, and placed apart.
2. At the point whilst the exhibit peruses HOT, encompass diced bacon and cook dinner for round 5 minutes till firm, mixing a good deal of the time.
3. Exchange the bacon to a paper towel-covered plate.
4. Add the meat to the pot in a solitary layer and cook for a couple of minutes to darker, at that point flip and rehash for the other facet.

5. Add onions and garlic. Cook for a few minutes to mellow, mixing regularly.
6. Include pink wine and tomato glue, making use of a wooden spoon to fast rub up tasty dark-colored bits adhered to the base of the pot.
7. Blend to watch that the tomato glue is damaged. Mood killer the sauté mode.
8. Exchange the hamburger back to the pot. Include mushrooms, carrots, and thyme, mixing collectively. Top with sound leaves.
9. Secure and seal the cover. Cook at a high weight for forty minutes, trailed through a manual weight discharge.
10. Reveal and pick out the sauté mode. Evacuate instantly leaves.
11. Give the stew a risk to bubble for a second to thicken at the same time as mixing. Mood killer the sauté mode. Serve into dishes and pinnacle with firm bacon.

Nutrition Information: Calories 220g, Fat 5g, Carb 6.5g, Sugars 2g, Protein 27g

Paleo Beef Barbacoa

Prep Time: 5mins, Cook Time: 1hr, Serving: 6, Point value: 4

Ingredients

- 3 - pounds grass-fed chuck roast fat
- 1 - large onion
- 6 - garlic cloves
- 2 4 -oz can of green chilis
- 1 - tablespoon oregano
- 1 - teaspoon salt
- 1 - teaspoons pepper
- 3 - dried chipotle peppers stems
- juice of 3 limes
- 3 - tablespoons coconut vinegar
- 1 - tablespoon cumin
- ¼ - cup water

Instructions

1. Add all fixings to the Instant Pot and mix.
2. Spot cover on, make sure the vent is shut and hit the "manual" seize. Increment time to an hour.
3. When executed, let generally discharge or press "drop" and discharge the load.
4. Evacuate top, shred with a fork, and hit the "sauté" seize. Blend mechanically because the juices lessen.
5. This might also take up to twenty-half-hour to completely lessen.

Nutrition Information: Calories 126g, Fat 5g, Carbs 4g, Sugar 2g, Protein 12g

Fall-Apart instant Pot Roast

Prep Time: 10mins, Cook Time, 1-hour 20mins, Serving: 3, Point value: 9

Ingredients

- 3 - lb grass-fed chuck roast, 1 - medium onion

- 2 - Tbsp. coconut oil, 1 - tsp. sea salt
- 2 - cups water or bone broth

Instructions

1. Turn Instant Pot to Sauté. Include the oil.
2. While shining, include the pot broil. Cook 2-3 minutes to brilliant; at that point flip to burn opposite side.
3. Sprinkle on the ocean salt. Top with cut onion. Pour in the water or juices.
4. Close and lock the top. Set Instant Pot to "Manual" and program for 70 minutes.
5. You may do fast discharge or characteristic discharge.

Nutrition Information: Calories 226g, Fat 15g, Carbs 1g, Sugar 0.5g, Protein 22g

Instant Pot Beef and Broccoli

Prep Time: 10mins, Cook Time: 30mins, Servings: 4, Point value: 8

Ingredients

- 1 ½ - pounds roast beef
- 12 - ounces broccoli florets
- 4 - cloves garlic minced
- 1 - tablespoon canola oil

For the sauce:
- ½ - cup beef broth
- ½ - cup low-sodium sauce
- ¼ - cup sweetener
- 1 - tablespoon corn starch

Instructions

1. Select the sauté mode at the weight cooker for medium warmth and encompass canola oil.
2. At the factor when the pot is hot, include garlic and cut hamburger.
3. Include hamburger juices, soy sauce, and sugar.
4. Blend together to interrupt up the sugar. Mood killer the sauté mode.
5. Secure and seal the top. Cook for 15 minutes at the excessive weight.
6. While striking tight for the load cooker, cook broccoli through microwaving for 3-4 minutes until sensitive.
7. At the point whilst the burden cooker is performed, bodily discharge weight through cautiously turning the discharge cope with its venting function.
8. Reveal the weight cooker and evacuate round 1/four measure of fluid.
9. Blend it with corn starch in a little bowl till absolutely broke down and clean, and add it back to the pot.
10. Give the sauce a chance to stew for around 5mins to thicken it relatively, blending regularly.
11. Add cooked broccoli again to the pot and fast combo to coat with the sauce.
12. Serve directly with an aspect, for instance, cauliflower rice.

Nutrition Information: Calories 310g, Fat 9g, Carb 10g, Sugars 4g, Protein 41g

Paleo Beef Brisket Pho an Instant Pot

Prep Time: 20mins, Cook Time: 40mins, Servings: 8, Point value: 9

Ingredients

- 1.75 - 2 lbs. Beef brisket
- 1-1.25 lbs beef shank soup bones
- 1 ¼ - cups dry shiitake mushrooms
- 3 - loose carrots
- 1 - medium size yellow onion
- 1 - large size leek
- Water
- 2 ½ - tsp fine sea salt
- 1 - tbsp Red Boat fish sauce
- 1 - tsp five spice powder
- Tea bags or cheese cloth

Pho Aroma Combo:
- 2 - fat thumb size ginger
- 4 - star anise
- 2 - cinnamon sticks
- 8 - green cardamom
- 3 - medium size shallots
- 4-5 - cilantro roots

Garnish:
- Lime wedges
- Baby bok choy
- Bean sprouts
- Red or green fresno chili peppers
- Mint leaves
- Asian/Thai basil
- Cilantro

Instructions

1. In a 6-quart estimate moment pot, include meat bones, brisket, diced carrots, odor mixture, and leeks. Strain the mushroom water as you upload the fluid to the pot. Fill the pot with extra faucet water until it achieves the 4-liter imprint. Close the quilt in Sealing function - Press Soup - Adjust to 40 mins/High weight/More.
2. Permit the moment pot come to feature weight discharge get rid of the whole onion and fragrance mixture in tea packs.
3. Evacuate the brisket and absorb it cold water for in any occasion 10 minutes. This will keep the beef from turning stupid shading. Dispose of fragrance and leek tea packs, yellow onion, and meat bones. Season the soup with 2 ½ tsp first-class ocean salt, 1 tbsp fish sauce, and 1 tsp 5 zest powder.

4. Flimsy reduce the brisket in 45-diploma factor and opposite to what might be predicted. Scoop the inventory over bean grows, carrots, mushrooms, mint leaves, Asian basil, stew peppers, and reduce brisket. Serve hot with lime wedges.

Nutrition Information: Calories 348g, Fat 7.1g, Carbs 34g, Sugar 3g, Protein 42g

Frozen Ground Beef in the Instant Pot

Prep Time: 1min, Cook Time: 25mins, Serving: 5, Point value: 13

Ingredients

- 2 - pounds ground beef, 1 - cup water

Instructions

1. Spot a trivet or steam crate inside the liner of your Instant Pot.
2. Include solidified ground meat top of the trivet, in one major square.
3. Include water underneath the trivet.
4. Lock the top, close the fixing valve, and select 25 minutes of weight cooking on high.
5. When the program is done, discharge the weight quickly by opening the valve.
6. Spot a towel over the valve to contain the steam and ensure your cabinets on the off chance that you like.
7. Take the temperature of your meat, utilizing a moment red meat thermometer. Go for 160F.
8. In the event that the meat is half-cooked, close the cover, seal, and cook for an additional 5 minutes checking once more.
9. Rehash if fundamental.
10. Expel ground hamburger with tongs. Utilize a tough spoon to disintegrate the ground meat.
11. Use in your preferred formula or stop the meat in pre-partitioned packs.

Nutrition Information: Calories 403g, Fat 13g, Carbs 11g, Sugar 3.2g, Protein 35g

Keto Low Carb Chili Recipe Instant Pot

Prep Time: 15mins, Cook Time: 8hrs, Serving: 2, Point value: 9

Ingredients

- 2 ½ - lb Ground beef
- ½ - large Onion
- 8 - cloves Garlic
- 2 15-oz can Diced tomatoes
- 1 6-oz can Tomato paste
- 1 4 -oz can Green chiles
- 2 - tbsp Worcestershire sauce
- ¼ - cup Chili powder
- 2 - tbsp Cumin

- 1 - tbsp Dried oregano
- 2 - tsp Sea salt
- 1 - tsp Black pepper
- 1 - medium Bay leaf

Instructions

1. Select the "Sauté" setting on the weight cooker. Include the cleaved onion and cook dinner for 5 -7mints, till translucent. Include the garlic and prepare dinner for a moment or less, until aromatic.
2. Include the ground meat. Cook for eight-10 minutes, breaking separated with a spatula until sautéed.
3. Include remaining fixings, except a valid leaf, to the Instant Pot and mix till consolidated. Spot the bay leaf into the center, if making use of.
4. Close the duvet. Press "Keep Warm/Cancel" to prevent the saute cycle. Select the "Meat/Stew" putting 35mins to start weight cooking.
5. Sit tight for the common discharge at the off chance that you could, or flip the valve to "vent" for speedy discharge if you're quick on agenda. On the off hazard which you applied a bay leaf, evacuate it earlier than serving.

Nutrition Information: Calories 265g, Fat 11g, Carbs 15g, Sugar 3g, Protein 23g

Meatballs in the Instant Pot

Prep Time: 15mins, Cooking Time: 15mins, Serving: 5, Point value: 20

Ingredients

For the meatballs:

- 1.5 - lbs ground beef
- 2 - Tbsp fresh parsley
- ¾ - cup grated parmesan cheese
- ½ - cup almond flour
- 2 - eggs
- 1 - tsp kosher salt
- ¼ - tsp ground black pepper
- ¼ - tsp garlic powder
- 1 - tsp dried onion flakes
- ¼ - tsp dried oregano
- 1/3 - cup warm water

To cook the meatballs:
- 1 - tsp olive oil
- 3 - cups easy keto marinara sauce

Instructions

1. Join meatball fixings in a medium bowl and blend altogether by hand.
2. Structure into around 15 two-inch meatballs.
3. Coat the base of the Instant Pot embed with the olive oil.

4. On the off chance that you wish to dark-colored them, turn on the saute capacity and darker on the two sides
5. Layer the seared or crude meatballs in the Instant Pot, leaving 1/2 inch of room between them. Try not to push down.
6. Pour the marinara sauce uniformly over the meatballs.
7. Seal the Instant Pot as indicated by the maker's guidelines.
8. Set the Instant Pot to Manual.

Nutrition Information: Calories 455g, Fat 33g, Carbs 5g, Sugar 2.3g, Protein 34g

Instant Pot Butter Beef

Prep Time: 10mins, Cook Time: 1hr, Servings: 6, Point value: 13

Ingredients

- 3 - lb beef roast such as a chuck
- 1 - tablespoon olive oil
- 2 - tablespoons ranch dressing seasoning mix
- 1 - pint jar pepper rings
- 2 - tablespoons zesty Italian seasoning mix
- 8 - tablespoons butter
- 1 - cup water

Instructions

1. Turn the Instant Pot or weight cooker to saute or dark colored. Spot the one tablespoon of olive oil in the base of the pot when it is hot. Since the two sides of the dish in the pot.
2. Turn the pot off and pour the water, flavoring blends, pepper rings, held squeezes over the meat cook. Spot the stick of spread over the dish.
3. Lock the cover onto the Instant Pot. Seal the valve. Physically set the ideal opportunity for an hour of weight. For bigger meals, it could take an hour and a half.
4. At the point when the cooking is finished, you can either take into account characteristic discharge or utilize the fast discharge. Cut up the hamburger with a plate of mixed greens sheers or break separated with forks.
5. Present with pureed cauliflower or pureed potatoes.

Nutrition Information: Calories 310.1, Fat 14.2g, Carbs 26.3g, Sugars 4.1g, Protein 3.8g

Cabbage Soup with Ground Beef Instant Pot

Prep Time: 15mins, Cook Time: 4hrs, Servings 1, Point value: 16

Ingredients

- 1 - tbsp Avocado oil
- 1 - large Onion
- 1 - lb Ground beef

- 1 - tsp Sea salt
- ¼ - tsp Black pepper
- 1 - lb Shredded coleslaw mix
- 1 15-oz can Diced tomatoes
- 6 - cups Beef bone broth
- 1 - tbsp Italian seasoning
- ½ - tsp Garlic powder
- 2 - medium Bay leaf

Instructions

1. Press the Sauté to seize at the Instant Pot. Include the oil and hacked onions. Cook for round 10-15 minutes, mixing by the way until onions begin to darker.
2. Add ground hamburger to the Instant Pot. Season with ocean salt and darkish pepper. Increment sautes temperature to "High". Cook, breaking separated with a spatula, for round 7-10 minutes, until the hamburger is cooked through.
3. At the point whilst the hamburger is performed, remodel off warm temperature and include the relaxation of the fixings into the Instant Pot. Blend to consolidate. Season with step by step salt and add pepper to flavor.
4. Spread and seal the Instant Pot. Press the Manual trap and modify the opportunity to 20mins. When cooking is completed, given weight a chance to discharge commonly for 5 minutes, at that factor utilizes snappy discharge. Evacuate the cove leaves before serving.

Nutrition Information: Calories 377g, Fat 26g, Carbs 2g, Sugar 1.2g, Protein 30g

Instant Pot Low-Carb Goulash Soup and Ground Beef with Peppers

Prep Time: 15mins, Cook Time: 15min, Serving: 6-8, Point value: 10

Ingredients:

- 1 ½ – 2 lbs. Extra lean ground beef
- 3 - tsp. olive oil
- 1 - large red bell pepper
- 1 - large onion
- 1 - T minced garlic
- 2 - T sweet paprika
- ½ - tsp. hot paprika
- 4 - cups homemade beef stock
- 14.5 oz. petite diced tomatoes
- sour cream for serving

Instructions

1. Turn the Instant Pot to sauté', heat the 2 tsp. olive oil, and cook the ground meat, breaking it separated with your fingers as you place it into the Instant Pot and furthermore with a turner as it cooks.
2. At the point when the meat is generally cooked, evacuate to a bowl
3. While the meat cooks, remove the stem and seeds from the red pepper and cut into off strips. Cut onion into off strips, the same size as the red pepper.

4. Include the other tsp. olive oil to the Instant Pot, include the onions and peppers and cook 3-4 minutes.
5. At that point include the minced garlic, sweet paprika, and hot paprika and cook 2-3 minutes longer; blending so the paprika is altogether cooked.
6. Include the hamburger stock or juices and petite diced tomatoes, alongside the ground meat.
7. Lock the top and utilize the SOUP setting, changing the opportunity to 15 minutes.
8. At the point when the cooking stops, let the weight discharge physically for a couple of minutes, at that point utilize brisk discharge to get done with discharging.
9. Serve hot with a liberal touch of harsh cream whenever wanted.

Nutrition Information: Calories 347g, Fat 21g, Carbs 8g, Sugar 1.3g, Protein 36g

Low-FODMAP Pressure Cooker Italian Beef

Prep Time: 15mins, Cooking Time: 2hs 35mins, Serving: 6, Point value: 18

Ingredients

- 5 - lbs. boneless beef roast
- 3 - tbsp garlic-infused olive oil
- 2 - tsp crushed red pepper
- 2 - tsp oregano
- 1 - tbsp basil
- 2 - tbsp pink Himalayan salt
- 1 - tbsp freshly cracked black pepper
- 1 32 oz jar Mezzetta Peperoncini
- 1 - cup beef broth, homemade or store-bought

Instructions

1. Utilizing a sharp serrated blade, cleave meat into 1-inch 3D shapes and spot away pack.
2. Include garlic-mixed olive oil and flavors to pack and delicately pivot the sack to convey the oil and flavors.
3. Spot stockpiling sack in the fridge and permit to marinate for at any rate 2 hours, ideally medium-term.
4. After marination of meat, pour a container of Mezzetta Peperoncini, hamburger, and meat juices into weight cooker embed.
5. Set Instant Pot to "Hamburger/Stew" and set the clock to 120 minutes.
6. After the weight cooker has finished the cooking procedure, enable it to normally depressurize for 20 minutes.
7. Following 20 minutes, turn the cover spout to completely depressurize.
8. Serve Italian Beef in dishes bested high with Mezzetta Peperoncini and appreciate

Nutrition Information: Calories 588g, Fat 28.8g, Carbs 3.3g, Sugar 1.4g, Protein 78.3g

Instant Pot Beef Stroganoff

Prep Time: 5mins, Cook Time: 30mins, Servings: 4, Point value: 11

Ingredients

- 1 - tablespoon oil
- ½ - cup diced onions
- 1 - tablespoon garlic
- 1 - pound beef stew meat
- 1.5 - cups chopped mushrooms
- 1 - tablespoon Worcestershire sauce
- 1 - teaspoon salt
- ½ -1 - teaspoon pepper
- ¾ - cup water

For Finishing:
- 1/3 - cup sour cream
- ¼ - teaspoon xanthum gum

Instructions

1. Turn Instant Pot on Sauté on outlandish, and when it is hot, encompass the oil.
2. At the factor, while the oil is warm, fuse onions and garlic and blend for a long time.
3. Fuse cheeseburger, mushrooms, Worcestershire sauce, salt, pepper, and water.
4. Close the weight cooker and set to 20 minutes on outlandish weight, Let it discharge weight by and large for 10 minutes.
5. By at that point, discharge any fingering weight.
6. Shake inside the xanthum gum a bit at some irregular moment, and continue mixing till the combo thickens.
7. In case you're utilizing corn starch, and so forth. blend a slurry with a bit water and use it to thicken.
8. Present with cauliflower rice or low carb noodles.

Nutrition Information: Calories 321g, Fat 16g, Carbs 9g, Sugar 3g, Protein 33g

Keto Instant Pot Chunky Chili

Prep Time: 10mins, Cook Time: 25mins, Servings: 2, Point value: 20

Ingredients

- 1 ¼ - lb ground beef
- 1 - tbsp olive oil
- ½ - medium sized yellow onion
- 2 - cloves garlic
- 1 ½ - tbsp chili powder
- 2 - tsp cumin
- 1 ½ - tsp sea salt

- 1 - tsp smoked paprika
- 1 - tsp garlic powder
- ¼ - tsp coriander powder
- ⅛ - tsp cayenne pepper
- 1 - cup beef broth
- ⅔ - cup water
- ¼ - cup canned pumpkin unsweetened kind
- 1 - cup canned diced tomatoes
- 2 - tbsp tomato paste
- ⅔ - cup cauliflower
- 1 - cup zucchini squash

Toppings:
- ⅔ - cup grated cheddar cheese
- ½ - of an avocado
- 3 - tbsp sour cream

Instructions

1. Select Saute and as soon as the Instant Pot is hot encompass olive oil and fall apart the ground meat into the pot. Sauté ground meat for 6 minutes, or till hamburger is carmelized while utilising a wooden spoon to mix and separate the hamburger.
2. When the hamburger has sautéed, encompass the cleaved onions and minced garlic and saute until translucent.
3. Include all of the relaxation of the fixings apart from the garnishes to the pot and mix to join.
4. Close and secure the cover and turn the load discharge take care of to the Sealing function. Select Pressure Cook on High Pressure and set the clock for 25 minutes.
5. When cooking time is completed, permit weight Naturally discharge for 10mins and later on carefully Quick Release all the relaxation of the burden. Give all of the weight a hazard to discharge.
6. Open the cover, combination and serve bested with cheddar, hacked avocado and a ½ tbsp of harsh cream or paleo acrid cream.

Nutrition Information: Calories 420g, Fat 32g, Carbs 8.5g, Sugars 3g, Protein 22g

★★ WW INSTANT POT DESSERT

Garlic Ginger Red Cabbage

Prep Time: 5mins, Cook Time: 10mins, Servings: 6, Point value: 3

Ingredients

- 2 - Tablespoons coconut oil
- 1 - Tablespoon butter
- 3 - cloves garlic crushed
- 2 - teaspoons fresh ginger grated
- 8 - cups red cabbage shredded
- 1 - teaspoon salt
- ½ - teaspoon pepper
- 1/3 - cup water

Instructions

1. Press the sauté capture and consist of the coconut oil and spread.
2. Whenever liquefied, include the garlic and ginger and blend properly.
3. Include your cabbage, salt, pepper, and water.
4. Close cover and lock the vent.
5. Press the guide capture and set for 5mins.
6. Fast discharge or discharge the burden typically when accomplished.
7. Blend nicely and serve.
8. To make at the stove.
9. Add cabbage to a microwave bowl and prepare dinner for five minutes.
10. In the meantime soften coconut oil and unfold in an large pot over medium-high warm temperature.
11. Include the garlic and ginger and sauté for a second or until aromatic.
12. Include the cabbage and half of the water, blend, and spread and flip the warm temperature down to medium.
13. Cook until the cabbage is as delicate as you might need.
14. Blend properly and serve.

Nutrition Information: Calories 56g, Fat 3g, Carbs 6g, Sugars 3g, Protein 1g

Instant Pot Keto Poblano Cheese Frittata

Prep Time: 10mins, Cook Time: 30mins, Serving: 4, Point value: 12

Ingredients

- 4 - eggs
- 1 - cup half and half
- 10 - ounce diced canned green chilies

- ½ -1 teaspoon salt
- ½ - teaspoon ground cumin
- 1 - cup Mexican blend shredded cheese
- ¼ - cup chopped cilantro

Instructions

1. Beat eggs and consolidate with creamer, diced green bean stews, salt, cumin, and 1/2 c of the destroyed cheddar.
2. Fill a 6-inch lubed metal or silicone dish, spread with foil. Make sure to oil the container well, since eggs stick it something furious.
3. Include some water into your Instant Pot, and spot a trivet in the pot. Spot the secured skillet on the trivet.
4. Cook at high weight for 20 minutes, permit characteristic discharge for 10 minutes and afterward discharge any residual weight.
5. Dissipate staying half measure of cheddar over the quiche, and spot under hot grill for 5mins until cheddar is percolating and dark colored.

Nutrition Information: Calories 257g, Fat 19g, Carbs 6g, Sugar 1.3g, Protein 14g

Simple Instant Pot Frittata

Prep Time: 45mins, Cooking Time: 1hr 5mins, Serving: 4, Point value: 3

Ingredients

- 6 - Eggs beaten
- ½ - cup Fresh Spinach chopped
- ¼ - cup Tomato diced
- 1 - tsp Sea Salt
- 1 - tsp Minced Onion
- ½ - tsp Garlic Powder
- ¼ - tsp Black Pepper

Instructions

1. Oil a container that fits within your instant pot. I utilize one of my tempered steel stackable instant pot dish however you can utilize a 7 in. Spring form, glass pyrex, or make it singular size in 4oz. Small scale bricklayer shakes also!
2. Mix the majority of the fixings together and add to your preparing vessel of decision. Spread with foil.
3. Add some water to your instant pot. Spot the dish containing your frittata blend over the trivet and painstakingly put this within your instant pot. Put the cover on and ensure the valve is in the sealing position.
4. Utilizing the showcase board selects the manual/pressure cook work. Utilize the +/ - catches to choose 5 minutes.
5. At the point when the pot is done cooking let it normally discharge the weight for 10 minutes. At that point flip the valve to the venting position and evacuate your frittata. Serve right away. Appreciate

Nutrition Information: Calories 82.9g, Fat 0.4g, Carbs 11.6g, Sugars 8.6g, Protein 9g

Instant Pot Bone Broth

Prep Time: 40mins, Cook Time: 4hrs, Servings: 24, Point value: 6

Ingredients

- 4 - lbs beef bones, 2 - tbsp Pink Himalayan Salt, water

Instructions

1. Preheat your stove to 400 degrees.
2. Add the defrosted issues that remain to be worked out the huge pot, load up with water and heat to the point of boiling, cooking for a sum of 20 minutes on the stove top. Skim off the stained froth that has amassed at the highest point of the water and channels the bones.
3. Wipe off the bones, in the event that any abundance froth buildup is on them and, at that point exchange to a huge heating sheet in a solitary layer. Cook for 20-25 minutes.
4. Expel the broiled bones and exchange to your moment pot. Deglaze the container with a sprinkle of water and scrape up any of the dark colored bits. Pour the bits and fat from the container over the bones in the moment pot.
5. Fill the pot with water, submerging every one of the bones. Include the salt and seal with the moment pot top.
6. Ensure your spout in on seal when cooking. Cook for 3-4 hours on manual weight.
7. Permit to rest 20 minutes before opening the moment pot. Strain the stock into an enormous bowl to take into account snappier cooling.
8. Add ice shapes to the stock or submerge the bowl into a huge ice shower. The stock should descend in temperature, cooling all things considered for 20 minutes.
9. Exchange the soup to bricklayer containers and seal firmly. Store in ice chest as long as 7 days or stop as long as 2 months.
10. Appreciate as a warm beverage or in plans

Nutrition Information: Calories 1g, Fat 0g, Carbs 0g, Sugars 0g, Protein 0g

Keto Instant Pot Blueberry Muffins

Prep Time: 30mins, Cooking Time: 55mins, Serving: 4, Point value: 6

Ingredients

- ⅓ - cup coconut flour
- 1 ½ - tbsp golden flaxseed meal
- 4 ½ - tbsp erythritol sweetener
- 1 - tsp baking powder
- ¼ - tsp baking soda
- ⅛ - tsp sea salt
- ⅓ - cup unsweetened almond milk

- 2 - large eggs, beaten
- 1 ½ - tbsp butter melted
- 1 - tsp vanilla extract
- ⅓ - cup fresh blueberries

Instructions

1. In a huge blending, bowl consolidates coconut flour, flaxseed dinner, erythritol sugar, heating powder, preparing soft drink and ocean salt. Blend and separate any bunches and put aside.
2. In a medium-sized blending, bowl joins almond milk, eggs, softened margarine, and vanilla concentrate. Blend altogether.
3. Add the wet blend to the dry blend and blend until cluster free. Delicately crease in the blueberries. Put aside.
4. Empty some water into the inward pot of the Instant Pot.
5. Fill six reusable silicone cupcake preparing liners ¾ of the route up with the biscuit player. The hitter is thick, and you should press the mixture down into the glasses with your fingers.
6. Spot a 10-inch sheet of tin foil over the steamer rack. Spot the biscuit glasses over the foil-arranged rack and overlap overabundance foil around the sides of the biscuits. Utilizing the rack handles, bring down the rack with the biscuits into the inward pot of the Instant Pot
7. Spot the second sheet of tin foil over the highest point of the biscuits to cover them. Close and lock the cover and turn the weight discharge handle to Sealing.
8. Select Pressure Cook on High Pressure and set the clock for 20 minutes.
9. When cooking time is finished, utilize the Natural Release strategy for 10 minutes and after that Quick Release the rest of the weight.
10. Open the top and evacuate tin foil spread. Utilizing the rack handles, lift the rack with biscuits out of the pot. Serve.

Nutrition Information: Calories 106.6g, Fat 1.3g, Carbs 20.8g, Sugars 8.2g, Protein 2.3g

---

Ropa Vieja Instant Pot

Prep Time: 10mins, Cooking Time: 15mins, Serving: 10, Point value: 12

Ingredients

- 3 – 3 ½ pound chuck roast
- 1 - onion
- 4 - teaspoons minced garlic
- 2 ½ - teaspoons dried oregano
- 2 - teaspoons cumin
- 2 - teaspoons paprika
- 2 - teaspoons salt
- 1 - teaspoon smoked paprika

- ½ - teaspoon black pepper
- ⅛ - teaspoon ground cloves
- 14.5 - ounce diced tomatoes
- 2 - bay leaves
- 3 - bell peppers
- Green olives with pimentos

Instructions

1. Add the majority of the fixings to an Instant Pot.
2. Secure the cover, close the valve and cook for an hour and a half.
3. Normally discharge weight.
4. Shred the meat utilizing two forks.
5. Press the sauté catch, include the chime peppers and cook for 4-5 minutes, or until delicate.
6. Mix in the green olives.

Nutrition Information: Calories 340.7g, Fat 18.2g, Carbs 9.3g, Sugars 3.5g, Protein 34.2g

Instant Pot Chili Verde

Prep Time: 15mins, Cook Time: 25mins, Servings: 4, Point value: 10

Ingredients

- 2 - pounds boneless skinless chicken thighs
- 12 - ounces tomatillos
- 8 - ounces poblano peppers
- 4 - ounces jalapeño peppers
- 4 - ounces onions
- ¼ - cup water
- 5 - cloves garlic
- 2 - teaspoons ground cumin
- 1 ½ - teaspoons salt

For finishing:
- ¼ - ounce chopped cilantro leaves
- 1 - tablespoon fresh lime juice

Instructions

1. Include tomatillos, poblanos, jalapeños, onions, and water to the weight cooker. Disseminate garlic, cumin, and salt on top. Ultimately, include chicken thighs. Secure and seal the top. Cook at a high weight for 15 minutes, trailed by a manual weight discharge. Reveal and exchange just the chicken to a cutting board. Cut into nibble estimated pieces. Put aside.
2. Add cilantro and lime juice to the weight cooker. Utilize a submersion blender or ledge blender to puree the blend.

3. Select the saute mode on the weight cooker for medium warmth. Return the chicken to the blend. Bubble for around 10 minutes to thicken the sauce, blending once in a while. Serve and trimming with extra cilantro.

Nutrition Information: Calories 310g, Fat 15g, Carb 10g, Sugars 4.5g, Protein 37g

Tomatillo Chili

Prep Time: 15mins, Cook Time: 35mins, Serving: 4, Point value: 15

Ingredients

- 1 - pound Ground beef
- 1 - pound Ground pork
- 3 - Tomatillos
- ½ - white onion
- 6 - oz Tomato paste
- 1 - tsp Garlic Powder
- 1 - Jalapeno Pepper
- 1 - tbsp Ground Cumin
- 1 - tbsp Chili Powder
- ¼ - 1 cup water
- Salt to taste

Instructions

1. Dark colored the hamburger and pork. I want to utilize the weight cooker for caramelizing to make it a one-pot dinner and just a single dish to wash!
2. Add every other fixing to the weight cooker: tomatillo, onion, tomato glue, garlic, jalapeno, cumin, stew powder, and water.
3. Utilize around 1 glass water, contingent upon the model of weight cooker you own. Thoroughly blend.
4. Close and secure weight cooker. Cook at a high weight for 35 minutes, at that point, expel from warmth to enable the strain to drop normally.
5. Fill in as-is or with low carb garnishes of your decision!

Nutrition Information: Calories 325g, Fat 23g, Carbs 6g, Sugars 3g, Protein 20g

★★ WW INSTANT POT KITCHEN STAPLE

Instant pot Garlic "Butter" Chicken Recipe

Prep Time: 5mins, Cook Time: 40mins, Serving: 4, Point value: 14, Ingredients

Ingredients

- 4 - chicken breasts
- ¼ - cup turmeric ghee
- 1 - teaspoon salt
- 10 - cloves garlic

Instructions

1. Add the chicken bosoms to the weight cooker pot.
2. Include the ghee, salt, and diced garlic to the weight cooker pot.
3. Set weight cooker on high weight for 35 minutes. Adhere to your weight cooker's directions for discharging the weight.
4. Shred the chicken bosom in the pot.
5. Present with extra ghee if necessary.

Nutrition Information: Calories 404g, Fat 21g, Carbs 3g, Sugar 0.3g, Protein 47g

Teri's instant pot Sausage and Peppers

Prep Time: 5mins, Cooking Time: 30mins, Serving: 5, Point value: 31

Ingredients

- 2 19-ounce packages Johnsonville Italian Sausage
- 4 - large green bell peppers
- 28 - ounce diced tomatoes
- 15 - ounce tomato sauce
- 1 - cup water
- 1 - tablespoon basil
- 2 - teaspoons garlic powder
- 1 - tablespoon Italian seasoning

Instructions

1. In the weight cooking pot, consolidate tomatoes, tomato sauce, water, basil, garlic powder, and Italian flavoring.
2. Add frankfurters to the sauce. Spot the peppers over the wiener, however, don't blend.
3. Lock cover set up and select High Pressure. Set clock for 25 minutes and press begin.
4. At the point when blare sounds turn off weight cooker and utilize a brisk weight discharge to discharge the weight.
5. At the point when the valve drops cautiously evacuate the cover.

Nutrition Information: Calories 570g, Fat 59g, Carbs 23g, Sugar 11g, Protein 44g

Low Carb Sugar Free instant pot Strawberry Cheesecake Recipe

Prep Time: 5mins, Cook Time: 20mins, Serving: 10, Point value: 15

Ingredients

- 8 -ounce blocks of full-fat cream cheese
- 2/3 - cup of any cup for cup sugar substitute
- 1 - tsp vanilla extract
- 2 - eggs, room temperature
- Hand full of fresh strawberries

Instructions

1. The oil within your spring structure skillet.
2. With a blender, mix the cream cheddar until it is totally smooth without any protuberances.
3. Include the sugar and vanilla concentrate to the cream cheddar. Mix until the fixings are simply joined.
4. Include the eggs each one in turn. Keep on blending until the eggs have been totally blended in.
5. Empty the player into the spring structure container. Spread the base and sides of the container firmly with one bit of foil to keep the water from spilling into the skillet.
6. Spot rack at the base of the weight cooker.
7. Add enough water to weight cooker pot to cover the base weight cooker pot by 1 inch. Lower spring structure container onto the rack.
8. Close the weight cooker and cook on high for 20 minutes.
9. Complete a characteristic discharge and enable the cheesecake to somewhat cool 15 or 20 minutes inside the weight cooker.
10. Cautiously evacuate the cheesecake cake. Give the cheesecake a chance to come to room temperature and after that expel the foil.
11. Spread the cheesecake with cling wrap and refrigerate for a few hours.
12. Just before serving, dice strawberries and sprinkle over the highest point of the cheesecake. Trimming with extra strawberry syrup or whipped cream whenever wanted.

Nutrition Information: Calories 277g, Fat 26g, Carbs 6g, Sugars 3g, Protein 5g

Keto Instant Pot Buffalo Chicken Cauliflower

Prep Time: 10mins, Cook Time: 5mins, Servings: 6, Point value: 15

Ingredients

- 1 - head 1 head cauliflower chopped
- 2 - cups cooked chicken cubed

- ½ - cup buffalo sauce
- ¼ - cup ranch dressing
- ½ - block cream cheese cubed
- 2 - cups shredded cheddar cheese
- salt & pepper to taste

Instructions

1. Include cauliflower, chicken, seasonings, wild ox sauce and farm dressing to the Instant Pot. Blend.
2. Cook utilizing the manual setting for 5 minutes.
3. Enable the Instant Pot to discharge weight.
4. Open and promptly mix in cream cheddar.
5. Once completely consolidated, including cheddar. Blend.
6. Warmth on KEEP WARM for 10 minutes.
7. Serve sprinkled with wild ox sauce and some green onion.

Nutrition Information: Calories 344g, Fat 24g, Carbs 7.7g, Sugars 3g, Protein 23g

Instant pot Keto Almond Carrot Cake

Prep Time: 10mins, Cook Time: 50mins, Serving: 6, Point value: 15

Ingredients

- 3 - eggs
- 1 - cup almond flour
- 2/3 - cup Swerve
- 1 - teaspoon baking powder
- 1.5 - teaspoons apple pie spice
- ¼ - cup coconut oil
- ½ - cup heavy whipping cream
- 1 - cup carrots shredded
- ½ - cup walnuts

Instructions

1. Combine all fixings using a hand blender, till the mixture is properly-fused, and appears cushioned.
2. This will protect the cake from being thick as almond flour desserts can in some instances be.
3. Fill the lubed skillet and spread the box with foil.
4. In the internal liner of your Instant Pot, place some water, and a steamer rack.
5. Spot the foil-secured cake on the trivet.
6. Press the CAKE capture and permit it to cook for 40 mins.
7. Enable the pressure to discharge typically for 10 mins.
8. Discharge ultimate weight.
9. Give it a risk to cool before icing with an icing of your selection or serve plain.

Nutrition Information: Calories 268g, Fat 25g, Carbs 6g, Sugar 1g, Protein 6g

Instant Pot Chicken Cacciatore

Prep Time: 20mins, Cooking Time: 15mins, Serving: 4, Point value: 4

Ingredients

- 4 - chicken thighs
- kosher salt and fresh pepper
- olive oil spray
- ½ - can Crushed tomatoes
- ½ - cup diced onion
- ¼ - cup diced red bell pepper
- ½ - cup diced green bell pepper
- ½ - teaspoon dried oregano
- 1 - bay leaf
- 2 - tablespoons chopped basil

Instructions

1. Press sauté at the Instant Pot, softly splash with oil and dark colored hen on the 2 facets a couple of minutes.
2. Shower with really more oil and include onions and peppers.
3. Sauté till mellow and great, 5 minutes.
4. Pour tomatoes over the chicken and veggies, consist of oregano, clove leaf, salt, and pepper, and provide it a fast blend and spread.
5. Cook high weight 25mins; everyday discharge.
6. Evacuate instantly leaf, beautify with parsley and serve over pasta, squash or something you wish

Nutrition Information: Calories 133g, Fat 3g, Carbs 10.5g, Sugar 5g, Protein 14g

Low Carb instant pot Pork Roast with Cauliflower Gravy

Prep Time: 15mins, Cooking Time: 7hrs 30Mins, Serving: 6, Point value: 17

Ingredients

- 1 - teaspoon Sea Salt
- ½ - teaspoon Black Pepper
- 4 - cups chopped cauliflower
- 1 - medium Onion
- 4 - cloves Garlic
- 2 - ribs celery
- 8 - ounces portabella mushrooms
- 2 - tablespoons Coconut Oil
- 2 - cups Water

Instructions

1. In the base of your weight cooker, place cauliflower, onion, garlic, celery, and water.
2. Top with pork dish and season with ocean salt and pepper.
3. Cook under strain for an hour and a half if your dish is solidified, an hour if totally defrosted.
4. Fast depressurize following fabricates headings.
5. Cautiously expel pork broil from the weight cooker and spot in a stove confirmation dish.
6. Heat at 400 degrees while setting up the sauce, this renders the fat and fresh up the edges of the pork to be progressively similar to as though it was moderate cooked.
7. Exchange cooked vegetables and soup to your blender and mix until smooth, put aside.
8. In your weight cooker cook mushrooms in coconut oil until delicate, approximately 3-5 minutes.
9. Add mixed vegetables and keep on cooking on the saute capacity until it is thickened as wanted.
10. Serve mushroom sauce over destroyed pork.

Nutrition Information: Calories 360g, Fat 27.7g, Carbs 6.3g, Sugars 2.6g, Protein 20.6g

Keto Salsa Chicken Recipe

Prep Time: 5mins, Cook Time: 30mins, Serving: 3, Point value: 7

Ingredients

- 2 - lbs boneless skinless chicken thighs
- 3 - tbsp taco seasoning
- Salt and pepper
- 4 - ounces cream cheese
- 1 - cup salsa mild
- ¼ - cup chicken broth

Instructions

1. Spot the chicken thighs in the base of the Instant Pot. Sprinkle with taco flavoring and somewhat extra salt and pepper.
2. Include the cream cheddar, salsa, and soup and lock the top into spot. Utilize the manual setting and set the Instant Pot on high for 20 minutes. When it's done the cooking, enable the strain to discharge normally for 15 minutes.
3. Utilize the vent to discharge any residual weight and after that evacuate the top. Evacuate the chicken to a plate and utilize a drenching blender to puree the sauce until smooth. On the other hand, you can exchange the sauce to a normal blender and puree.
4. Shred the chicken with two forks and include once more into the pot. Hurl to coat in the smooth sauce. Present with lettuce wraps and top with cleaved avocados and destroyed cheddar.

Nutrition Information: Calories 244g, Fat 9.9g, Carbs 4.2g, Sugar 1g, Protein 30.2g

Instant Pot Keto Breakfast Casserole

Prep Time: 10mins, Cook Time: 42mins, Servings: 6, Point value: 17

Ingredients

- 2 - tbsp avocado oil
- 6 - ounces breakfast sausage
- 3 - medium broccoli stalks
- 2 - garlic cloves minced
- Salt and pepper
- 6 - large eggs
- ¼ - cup heavy cream
- 1 - cup Monterey Jack cheese
- 1 - green onion thinly
- 1 - California Avocado
- Salsa, additional cheese

Instructions

1. Oil a 7-inch distance across meal dish or souffle dish.
2. Turn the Instant Pot onto the sauté capacity and include the avocado oil. When hot, include the mass hotdog and split it up with a wooden spoon. Cook around 4 minutes until the majority of the pink is no more.
3. Include the ground broccoli stalks, garlic, and salt and pepper. Keep on cooking an additional 2 minutes until the broccoli is delicate. Exchange the blend to the readied preparing dish.
4. In a medium bowl, whisk together the eggs and cream until very much consolidated. Mix in the cheddar and the green onion. Pour over the hotdog blend in the dish. Spread the dish firmly with aluminum foil
5. Empty some water into the base of the Instant Pot and include the trivet. Spot the dish over the trivet and lock the cover. Ensure the vent is shut. Set the cooker to manual weight for 35 minutes.
6. At the point when the cooking cycle is finished, given the weight a chance to discharge normally for 10 minutes. At that point vent until all the weight is no more.
7. Top the dish with the meagerly cut avocado before serving. Top with some other fixings you want.

Nutrition Information: Calories 351g, Fat 28.5g, Carbs 6.8g, Sugar 2.1g, Protein 18.6g

INSTANT POT LEMON GARLIC SALMON

Prep Time: 3mins, Cook Time: 17mins, Serving: 4, Point value: 11

Ingredients

- 1 ½ - pounds frozen salmon filets
- ¼ - cup lemon juice
- ¾ - cup water

- A few springs of fresh dill, basil
- ¼ - teaspoon garlic powder
- ¼ - teaspoon sea salt or to taste
- 1/8 - teaspoon black pepper
- 1 - lemon, sliced thinly
- 1 - tablespoon avocado oil

Instructions

1. Empty water and lemon juice into your Instant Pot. Add new herbs to the water/lemon juice blend and spot steamer rack in Instant Pot.
2. Sprinkle salmon with oil and season with salt and pepper.
3. Sprinkle garlic powder over the salmon and spot on the salmon in a solitary layer on the steamer rack in the Instant Pot.
4. Layer lemon cuts over the salmon.
5. Spot the cover on the Instant Pot, lock set up and turns the valve to fixing.
6. The utilization of the Manual setting to cook on HIGH weight for 7 minutes.
7. It will take your Instant Pot around 10 minutes to get up to weight.
8. When the time is up, change the valve to venting to snappy discharge the weight
9. Appreciate warm over a serving of mixed greens, with broiled veggies or whatever other way that you can cook up

Nutrition Information: Calories 296g, Fat 15g, Carbs 8g, Sugars 4g, Protein 31g

★★ WW INSTANT POT SNACK

Meatballs in the Instant Pot

Prep Time: 15mins, Cooking Time: 45mins, Serving: 3, Point value: 20

Ingredients

For the meatballs:

- 1.5 - lbs ground beef
- 2 - Tbsp fresh parsley
- ¾ - cup parmesan cheese
- ½ - cup almond flour
- 2 - eggs
- 1 - tsp kosher salt
- ¼ - tsp ground black pepper
- ¼ - tsp garlic powder
- 1 - tsp dried onion flakes
- ¼ - tsp dried oregano
- 1/3 - cup warm water
- **To cook the meatballs:**
- 1 - tsp olive oil
- 3 - cups keto marinara sauce

Instructions

1. Consolidate meatball fixings in a medium bowl and blend altogether by hand.
2. Structure into roughly 15 two-inch meatballs.
3. Coat the base of the Instant Pot embed with the olive oil.
4. In the event that you wish to dark-colored them, turn on the saute capacity and darker on the two sides – or dark colored in a different nonstick dish first.
5. Layer the caramelized or crude meatballs in the Instant Pot, leaving 1/2 inch of room between them. Try not to push down.
6. Pour the marinara sauce equitably over the meatballs.
7. Seal the Instant Pot as indicated by the maker's directions.
8. Set the Instant Pot to Manual.
9. Select low weight. Set the cooking time to 10 minutes.
10. When the clock goes off turn the valve to vent and enable the steam to disperse totally.
11. Expel the cover and serve the meatballs with sauce over zoodles or spaghetti squash whenever wanted.

Nutrition Information: Calories 455g, Fat 33g, Carbs 5g, Sugar 3g, Protein 34g

Instant Pot Low Carb Pizza Casserole

Prep Time: 15mins, Cooking Time: 25mins, Serving: 4, Point value: 36

Ingredients

- 2 - cups crushed tomatoes
- 1 - lbs ground turkey
- 1 - package pepperoni
- ½ - cup mozzarella cheese
- ½ - cup cheddar cheese
- 1 - tbsp oregano
- ½ - tsp salt
- 2 - clove minced garlic
- ½ - tsp pepper
- ½ - tsp onion powder

Instructions

1. Turn your IP on sauté mode. Include a teaspoon of olive oil. When warm, including ground turkey.
2. Season with salt, pepper, and half teaspoon garlic powder. Cook turkey altogether.
3. When performed, evacuate floor turkey and see in a special holder.
4. Wash out your IP liner with heated water.
5. Layer the fixings into a 7 field Pyrex dish: Pour 1/4 of the smashed tomatoes on the base of the Instant Pot.
6. At that point layer 1/four of the floor turkey, cheddar, and pepperoni on pinnacle.
7. Keep on layering pulverized tomatoes, floor turkey, cheddar, and pepperoni inside the Instant Pot. Make 3-4 layers
8. Spot some water into IP liner, place trivet at the bottom of your IP pot liner put Pyrex at the trivet.
9. Spot a piece of foil on top to prevent any fluids from falling into the dish.
10. Put on High guide weight for 20 minutes, and permit NPR for 15 minutes.
11. Expel the pinnacle and allow cool for 15 minutes to settle before reducing and serving.

Nutrition Information: Calories 554g, Fat 70g, Carbs 60g, Sugars 20g, Protein 30g

Instant pot Bruschetta Chicken with Zoodles

Prep Time: 15mins, Cook Time: 4mins, Servings: 4, Point value: 27

Ingredients

- 2 - pounds Chicken Breasts Boneless
- 2.5 - pounds Diced Tomatoes drained
- ½ - cup Red Onion diced
- 2/3 - cup Real/Fresh Parmesan Cheese shredded
- ¼ - cup Extra Virgin Olive Oil
- 2 - Tablespoons Balsamic Vinegar
- 1 - head Fresh Garlic peeled, minced
- 1 - Tablespoon Better than Bouillon Chicken Base

- ½ - teaspoon Sea Salt
- ¼ - teaspoon Freshly Ground Black Pepper
- ½ - cup Fresh Basil Leaves
- 2 - Tablespoons Butter
- 6-8 - ounces Mozzarella Cheese
- Zucchini

Instructions

1. Incorporate Chicken and Parmesan Cheese.
2. Lock on Lid and close Pressure Valve.
3. Cook at Low Pressure for 3 minutes.
4. Right when Beep sounds, grant a 5-minute typical weight release.
5. Open top and mix in Butter and Fresh Basil.
6. Spot Chicken on Zoodles or Pasta.

Nutrition Information: Calories 698g, Fat 39g, Carbs 18g, Sugars 9g, Protein 66g

Keto Instant Pot spice cake

Prep Time: 20mins, Cooking Time: 25mins, Serving: 3, Point value: 13

Ingredients

- 2 - cups almond flour
- ½ - cup erythritol
- 2 - tsp baking powder
- 1 - tsp ground cinnamon
- 1 - tsp ground ginger
- ¼ - tsp ground cloves
- ¼ - tsp salt
- 2 - large eggs
- 1/3 - cup butter, melted or coconut oil
- 1/3 - cup water
- ½ - tsp vanilla extract
- 3 - tbsp chopped toasted pecans or walnuts

Instructions

1. Oil a 7-inch artistic container well a soufflé dish works incredibly.
2. Spot the trivet in the base of the Instant Pot and include some water.
3. In an enormous bowl, whisk together the flour, sugar, preparing powder, cinnamon, ginger, cloves, and salt. Mix in the eggs, dissolved spread, water, and vanilla concentrate until very much consolidated.
4. Spread the hitter in the readied heating skillet and smooth the top. Sprinkle with slashed nuts. Spread the dish firmly with aluminum foil. Set over the trivet in the Instant Pot.
5. Close the cover and pick the cake setting. It will consequently set for 40 minutes. When the cycle is done, enable the Instant Pot to normally discharge the weight for 15

minutes. At that point evacuate the top and lift out the fired dish. Cool totally in the container.

6. Evacuate the foil and exchange the cake to a serving platter. Serve alone or with daintily improved whipped cream.

Nutrition Information: Calories 236g, Fat 23g, Carbs 5g, Sugar 2.1g, Protein 5g

Pecan Pie Cheesecake - Instant Pot Recipe

Prep Time: 25mins, Cook Time: 3hrs 35mins, Serving: 10, Point value: 19

Ingredients

Crust:

- ¾ - cup almond flour
- 2 - tbsp Swerve Sweetener
- Pinch salt
- 2 - tbsp melted butter

Pecan Pie Filling:

- ¼ - cup butter
- 1/3 - cup Swerve Sweetener
- 1 - tsp Yacon syrup
- 1 - tsp caramel extract
- 2 - tbsp heavy whipping cream
- 1 - large egg
- ¼ - tsp salt
- ½ - cup chopped pecans

Cheesecake Filling:

- 12 - ounces cream cheese
- 5 - tbsp Swerve Sweetener
- 1 - large egg
- ¼ - cup heavy whipping cream
- ½ - tsp vanilla extract

Topping:

- 2 - tbsp butter
- 2 ½ - tbsp Swerve Sweetener
- ½ - tsp Yacon syrup
- ½ - tsp caramel extract
- 1 - tbsp heavy whipping cream
- Whole toasted pecans for garnish

Instructions

1. In a medium bowl, whisk on the whole the almond flour, sugar, and salt. Mix inside the melted margarine till the blend begins off-developed to group together.

2. Press into the most reduced and halfway up the edges of a 7-inch springform field. Spot in the cooler while making the pecan pie filling.

3. Pecan Pie Filling:
4. In a clue pot over low warmth, soften the spread. Incorporate the sugar and Yacon syrup and race until joined, at that figure blend the paid intrigue and immense whipping cream.
5. Include the egg and hold cooking over low warmth till the blend thickens. Rapidly oust from the warm temperature and mix inside the pecans and salt.
6. Region mixed over the base of the outside layer.
7. Cheesecake Filling:
8. Beat the cream cheddar till simple, at that segment beat inside the sugar. Beat inside the egg, whipping cream, and vanilla a concentrate.
9. Pour this blend over the pecan pie filling and spread to the edges.
10. Wrap the base of the springform skillet solidly in a broad piece of foil. Recognize a piece of paper towel over the best factor of the springform skillet and after that overlay foil over the apex as well. Your total dish should be for the most extreme component covered in foil to keep out bounty clamminess.
11. Detect the rack that pursued your Instant Pot or weight cooker into the base. Void some water into the base.
12. Circumspectly decline the wrapped cheesecake field onto the rack.
13. Close the spread and set the Instant Pot to manual mode for 30 minutes on high. At the point when the cooking time is done, let the worry to release regularly.
14. Lift out the cheesecake and license it cool to room temperature, and after that refrigerate for 3 or 4 hours or even medium-timespan.
15. in a clue pot over low warm temperature, diminish the margarine. Incorporate the sugar and yacon syrup and speed till merged, by then blend inside the tune in and huge whipping cream.
16. Wash over the chilled cheesecake and improvement with toasted pecans.

Nutrition Information: Calories 340g, Fat 31.03g, Carbs 4.97g, Sugar 2.3g, Protein 5.89g

CONCLUSION

Thank you for downloading this book!

You will get an effective method for weight loss, healthy living while saving money.

I hope this book will help you to lose weight! If you enjoyed this book, would you be kind enough to share this book with your family, friends, and or co-workers and leave a review on Amazon. By you leaving an honest review for this book on Amazon you will help guide people on Amazon to know that this book is legit and perhaps it can help them out as well.

CPSIA information can be obtained
at www.ICGtesting.com
Printed in the USA
LVHW011106200221
679496LV00008B/92